Study Guide for the Licensed Practical/Vocational Hospice and Palliative Nurse

Editor
Tami Borneman, RN, PHN, MSN, CNS, FPCN
Advanced Practitioner
City of Hope National Medical Center
Department of Nursing Research & Education
Duarte, CA

HPNA
Hospice and Palliative Nurses Association

Kendall Hunt
publishing company

Development of this Study Guide

has been made possible by the

Hospice and Palliative Nurses Association

Revised printing 2010

ISBN 978-0-7575-2002-0

Printed in the United States of America
10 9 8 7 6 5

CONTENTS

Contributors

Tami Borneman, RN, PHN, MSN, CNS, FPCN
Advanced Practitioner
City of Hope National Medical Center
Department of Nursing Research & Education
Duarte, CA

Mary Ersek, PhD, RN, FAAN, FPCN
Associate Director
John A. Hartford Center of Geriatric Nursing Excellence and Center for Integrative Science in Aging

Associate Professor
University of Pennsylvania
School of Nursing
Philadelphia, PA

Linda Gorman, RN, MN, APRN, BC, OCN, CHPN®
Palliative Care/Hospice Clinical Nurse Specialist
Cedars Sinai Medical Center
Los Angeles, CA

Lynda Gruenewald-Schmitz, RN, MSN
Manager/Administrator
Aurora VNA Zilber Family Hospice
Wauwatosa, WI

Barbara Anderson Head, PhD, RN, CHPN®, ACSW
Faculty Researcher
University of Louisville School of Nursing
Louisville, KY

Judy Lentz, RN, MSN, NHA
Chief Executive Officer
Hospice and Palliative Nurses Association
Pittsburgh, PA

Jeanne Martinez, RN, MPH, CHPN®, FPCN
Quality Specialist, Palliative Care & Home Hospice
Northwestern Memorial Hospital
Chicago, IL

Beverly Paukstis, RN, MS, CHPN®, CHPCA®
Manager/Administrator
Community Hospice of DC
Washington, DC

Marty Richards, MSW, LICSW
Social Worker
Private Practice
Port Townsend, WA

Dena Jean Sutermaster, RN, MSN, CHPN®
Director of Education Products
Hospice and Palliative Nurses Association
Pittsburgh, PA

Christy Torkildson, RN, PHN, MSN
Manager/Administrator
Lead Instructor, Department of Nursing
Unitek College
San Francisco, CA

Sarah A. Wilson, PhD, RN
Associate Professor
Marquette University
Milwaukee, WI

Content Reviewers

Eileen Bennett, RN, BSN, OCN, CHPN®
Nurse Manager
Wellmont Hospice
Bristol, TN

Sue Boederker, RN, BSN, MSN
ADN Instructor
Gateway Technical College
Burlington, WI

Carole Heaney, RN, MSN
Vice President of Operations
The Community Hospice, Administrative Offices
Rensselaer, NY

Linda F. Hill, LPN
Hospice of Naples
Naples, FL

Kathleen Lavorgna, LPN, CHPLN®
Administrator
Gem City Home Care
Dayton, OH

Douglas Nee, PharmD, MS
Clinical Specialist/Consultant
Pain Management & Palliative Care
DR-Scripts, Inc.
San Diego, CA

Carol Shenise, MS, RN
Education Specialist
The Community Hospice, Inc.
Rensselaer, NY

Pam Stephenson, RN, MSN, CS, AOCN
Clinical Nurse Specialist
Hope Center for Cancer Care
Warren, OH

Kay Terry, RN, MSN, APRN
Nurse Practitioner
Care Source
Salt Lake City, UT

Tanya Walakovits, LPN
Home Care LPN
Capital Hospice
Washington, DC

Lana Walsh, LPN
Hospice of Naples
Naples, FL

Leslie Weichsel, MSN, APRN, BC
Chief Operating Officer
Hospice, Inc.
Poughkeepsie, NY

Disclaimer

The Hospice and Palliative Nurses Association, its officers and directors, and the authors and reviewers of this Study Guide make no claims that buying or studying it will guarantee a passing score on the CHPLN® Certification examination.

Introduction

HPNA recognizes the significant contribution to end-of-life care that is provided by licensed practical/vocational nurses (LP/VNs). As part of the interdisciplinary care team, they provide much needed care to the patients and their family members, promoting quality of life throughout the illness trajectory, the patient's death and family bereavement. To this end, HPNA is committed to developing educational products for HPNA LP/VN members. This is why the *Core Curriculum for the Licensed Practical/Vocational Hospice and Palliative Nurse* and *Study Guide for the Licensed Practical/Vocational Hospice and Palliative Nurse* have been created.

The study guide is divided into two sections by content areas. The first section includes questions that cover the scope of the licensed practical/vocational hospice and palliative nurse in the areas of physical, spiritual, psychosocial, and emotional care. The second section includes case studies that can be answered by an individual or used in a study group. Both the questions and case studies are followed by explanations of the answers. The case studies may also have other answers than those listed in this book.

This study guide is aimed at both experienced LP/VNs and those new to palliative care. We welcome your feedback on whether this study guide meets your needs and if you have other ideas for educational product development for LP/VNs. We strive to provide useful and pertinent information to promote excellence in hospice and palliative care across all levels of nursing in all settings of care.

Editor's Comments

Those of us who work in hospice and palliative nursing are ever aware of the unique and valuable contribution of the LP/VNs who provide hands-on care and compassionate support to patients at the end of life. It is a very special person who can attend to the personal care needs of patients whose physical condition is declining while emotional and spiritual needs may be escalating. The job can be physically demanding and emotionally draining, but day after day, you are at the bedside of those facing the challenges of terminal illness. Your work as part of the interdisciplinary team is very important and is to be commended.

It has indeed been an honor to assist with this project. My hope is that this guide will be a learning tool for all LP/VNs and will help build the confidence and knowledge needed for the process. Questions were developed based upon the *Core Curriculum for the Licensed Practical/Vocational Hospice and Palliative Nurse* and the test content outline was developed by the National Board for Certification of Hospice and Palliative Nurses (NBCHPN®). Some questions may seem challenging, but the intent is to stimulate learning about the various content areas. Case studies are given for the purpose of exploring and thinking through situations common to hospice and palliative care. Nurse practice acts for LP/VNs vary across the country and some information in this study guide may not be applicable to all LP/VNs. Medication names utilize "tall man" lettering where recommended by the Federal Drug Administration (FDA). To help differentiate between drug names that are similar, the FDA has suggested capitalizing a portion of the generic name. For example the generic name for Wellbutrin® is buPROPion.

Thanks to all the professionals who contributed questions and case studies to this guide and to the expert reviewers who gave of their time and talent. I think I can speak for all of us in saying that we are very proud to contribute to the process of assuring that hospice and palliative LP/VNs receive the much deserved credit and affirmation for the skills and knowledge they have and utilize to make life's end one of comfort and meaning for their patients and families. I wish you success.

Tami Borneman, RN, PHN, MSN, CSN, FPCN
Advanced Practitioner
City of Hope National Medical Center
Department of Nursing Research & Education
Duarte, CA

Study Questions and Answers

Interdisciplinary Team

1. Core members of the hospice team include which of the following?

   A. Licensed practical/vocational nurse, social worker, chaplain, registered nurse

   B. Registered nurse, social worker, counselor, physician

   C. Physician, dietitian, nursing assistant, registered nurse

   D. Registered nurse, licensed practical/vocational nurse, social worker, bereavement coordinator

2. The main difference between the multidisciplinary team and interdisciplinary team is

   A. Multidisciplinary teams are more common in hospice and interdisciplinary teams are more common in other settings

   B. The physician is a member of multidisciplinary teams but not of interdisciplinary teams

   C. The interdisciplinary team is used in the hospice setting and the multidisciplinary team is utilized in the palliative care setting

   D. The interdisciplinary team is used in the hospice setting and the multidisciplinary team is more common in the acute hospital non-palliative care setting

3. Which statement reflects the best way to enhance team collaboration?

   A. Team members submit written reports before the meeting to be read by the leader

   B. Team ground rules include that the leader makes final decision when there is a disagreement on the treatment plan

   C. Joint visits between the registered nurse, licensed practical/vocational nurse, and social worker are encouraged

   D. The physician and registered nurse develop the plan of care

1. Answer is B

   A. Incorrect: Licensed practical/vocational nurses and chaplains are valuable members of the interdisciplinary team, but are not core members according to federal regulations.

   B. **Correct:** Federal hospice regulations mandate hospices have these members of the core team.

   C. Incorrect: Dietitians and nursing assistant are valuable members of the interdisciplinary team, but are not core members according to federal regulations.

   D. Incorrect: Licensed practical/vocational nurses and bereavement coordinators are valuable members of the interdisciplinary team, but are not core members according to federal regulations.

2. Answer is D

   A. Incorrect: Interdisciplinary teams are seen more in hospice.

   B. Incorrect: There should be a physician member of both a multidisciplinary and interdisciplinary team. The physician is often the team leader of the multidisciplinary team.

   C. Incorrect: Hospice and palliative care utilize the interdisciplinary model.

   D. **Correct:** Multidisciplinary teams are teams where various members report on their progress with the patient. Hospice and palliative care promote more interaction between team members rather than just reporting. Physicians are generally members of the interdisciplinary in palliative care and always in hospice.

3. Answer is C

   A. Incorrect: Written reports do not promote collaboration.

   B. Incorrect: All involved in the decision-making process rather than just one or two people.

   C. **Correct:** Team collaboration is enhanced by involvement of different disciplines.

   D. Incorrect: Each discipline contributes to the plan of care.

4. Which statement about interdisciplinary team conflict is **NOT** true?

   A. A conflict can be a sign of professional growth as a team

   B. Role ambiguity can contribute to conflict

   C. Too large of a group for its function can increase conflict

   D. The presence of ground rules tends to breed resentment and increases conflict

5. Which of the following best reflects a key characteristic of the interdisciplinary team leader?

   A. In a true collaboration there is no need for an identified leader

   B. In hospice, the leader should be the registered nurse and in palliative care the leader should be a physician

   C. Any discipline can potentially be an effective leader

   D. The leader needs to have line management authority

6. Evaluation of the team process can be accomplished by

   A. Inviting the patient/family to the meeting to share insights

   B. Patient/family satisfaction surveys

   C. The administrator interviews the team leader to get a report on team functioning

   D. No evidence of conflict indicates the team is functioning effectively

4. Answer is D

A. Incorrect: Conflict is expected to occur since members are interdependent on each other.

B. Incorrect: Conflict can arise when team members are not clear on their and each other's roles.

C. Incorrect: Having too many people than are needed for a purpose can increase conflict.

D. **Correct:** Ground rules have been found to be a way to establish clear expectations for all members and can be very useful for a well-functioning team.

5. Answer is C

A. Incorrect: It is important to designate a team leader.

B. Incorrect: The team leader may be any member of the team.

C. **Correct:** The team leader is a key person who often sets the tone for the team functioning. Of less importance is the title or job description of the leader. More important is the skill in collaboration and communication. An identified leader tends to be helpful to keep things on track.

D. Incorrect: The team leader may be any member of the team.

6. Answer is B

A. Incorrect: Inviting the patient/family to the meeting to share insights is not an objective measure.

B. **Correct:** Patient/family satisfaction surveys provide an objective tool.

C. Incorrect: "The administrator interviews the team leader to get a report on team functioning" is not an objective measure.

D. Incorrect: Conflict can sometimes be hidden and expressed in other ways outside of the team meeting.

7. Which of the following statements best describes the licensed practical/vocational nurse role in the interdisciplinary team?

   A. Reports on physical and psychosocial assessments

   B. Attends the interdisciplinary team, but the registered nurse reports all nursing data

   C. Provides information as appropriate to the development of the plan of care

   D. Is designated to present the patient's voice

8. Which of the following is a **TRUE** statement about team functioning?

   A. Communication remains the most important activity

   B. Team leaders always determine the communication style of the team

   C. The team decides if it will be interdisciplinary or multidisciplinary

   D. Criticism of the team process is the role of the leader

9. Decisions made about patients receiving hospice or palliative care

   A. Need to be coordinated with all disciplines

   B. Can be made initially before all pertinent information has been collected if needed

   C. Should be made by the team leader

   D. Do not require knowledge of patient/family wishes

7. Answer is C

   A. Incorrect: Assessments of physical and psychosocial problems are done by the registered nurse.

   B. Incorrect: The licensed practical/vocational nurse should be encouraged to report on data observed.

   C. **Correct:** The licensed practical/vocational nurse as an important member of the team provides important information on the plan of care in conjunction with other team members.

   D. Incorrect: All team members should be expressing the patient's concerns.

8. Answer is A

   A. **Correct:** Communication between team members remains the key element to determine the effective functioning of the team.

   B. Incorrect: "Team leaders always determine the communication style of the team" does not describe effective team functioning.

   C. Incorrect: The purpose of the team dictates interdisciplinary or multidisciplinary teams.

   D. Incorrect: "Criticism of the team process is the role of the leader" does not describe effective team functioning.

9. Answer is A

   A. **Correct:** Coordinating decisions with all disciplines is a hallmark of hospice and palliative care.

   B. Incorrect: Decisions made must be based on input from the patient and appropriate family members. Some assessments of the patient's needs must be completed before contemplating care decisions.

   C. Incorrect: Coordinating decisions with all disciplines is a hallmark of hospice and palliative care.

   D. Incorrect: Decisions made must be based on input from the patient and appropriate family members.

10. Which of the following statements best describes signs of a well-functioning, interdisciplinary team?

A. Members never miss a meeting and rarely openly disagree

B. Members attend most meetings and actively participate in each meeting attended

C. Members disagree openly and the team leader makes final decisions in complex cases

D. The written plan of care is completed by the patient care coordinator and the physician reviews the document

Disease Progression

11. The most common sites of metastases are bone and

A. Bone marrow

B. Lung

C. Brain

D. Bowel

12. One of the chief psychosocial issues for people with lung cancer might be

A. Sadness over impending treatments

B. Fear of losing the ability to speak

C. Anger over medical mismanagement

D. Guilt due to smoking

10. Answer is B

   A. Incorrect: Absence of open conflict does not necessarily mean the team is functioning effectively.

   B. **Correct:** Characteristics of an effective team include collaboration between all members.

   C. Incorrect: One person from the team is never charged with making decisions.

   D. Incorrect: One or two persons from the team are never charged with developing the plan of care.

Disease Progression

11. Answer is B

   A. Incorrect: Bone marrow is not one of the most common metastatic sites.

   B. **Correct:** Lung is one of the most common metastatic sites.

   C. Incorrect: Brain is not one of the most common metastatic sites.

   D. Incorrect: Bowel is not one of the most common metastatic sites.

12. Answer is D

   A. Incorrect: Sadness over impending treatments is not one of the chief psychological issues for people with lung cancer.

   B. Incorrect: Fear of losing the ability to speak is not one of the chief psychological issues for people with lung cancer.

   C. Incorrect: Anger over medical mismanagement is not one of the chief psychological issues for people with lung cancer.

   D. **Correct:** Guilt about smoking and fear of suffocating are the chief psychological concerns of people with lung cancer.

13. Which of the following is a **TRUE** statement about cancer? It is a condition

    A. From which there is no expectation of cure

    B. Wherein the organs are invaded by bacteria

    C. Wherein cells lose their normal controls and traits

    D. Wherein the body systems become immune

14. A person with head and neck cancer who is receiving chemotherapy asks the nurse, "When I finish these treatments, will I be cured?" The best answer would be

    A. "What has the physician told you?"

    B. "Have you read anything about it on the Internet?"

    C. "Are you afraid of dying?"

    D. "How do you feel about the treatments?"

15. When caring for a person with brain cancer, the nurse needs to remember that one of the following symptoms may occur and needs to be monitored closely

    A. Seizures

    B. Bleeding

    C. Hemoptysis

    D. Dyspnea

13. Answer is C

A. Incorrect: With treatment, approximately 50% of cancers are cured.

B. Incorrect: Cancer is not a bacterium.

C. **Correct:** Cancer causes cells to lose their normal controls and traits.

D. Incorrect: The immune system attempts to rid the body of the cancer cells.

14. Answer is D

A. Incorrect: Asking about conversations with the physician will not get to the root of the patient's concerns.

B. Incorrect: Though it is important to know what a patient knows about their condition, asking what they have read on the Internet will not determine why they are asking this question.

C. Incorrect: While the person may be afraid of dying, you should let the patient bring this up first.

D. **Correct:** Asking the patient how they are feeling about their treatment is an open ended question designed to allow the patient to talk more about what their concerns are.

15. Answer is A

A. **Correct:** Seizures are a symptom of brain cancer.

B. Incorrect: Bleeding is not a symptom of brain cancer.

C. Incorrect: Hemoptysis is not a symptom of brain cancer.

D. Incorrect: Dyspnea is not a symptom of brain cancer.

16. Which of the following statements is **TRUE** about chemotherapy? It

   A. Can take the place of blood transfusions

   B. Always holds out false hope to people

   C. Can be used in palliative care

   D. Is always expensive but worth it

17. When caring for a person with AIDS, the nurse's teaching should begin with

   A. The signs of infection

   B. Universal precautions

   C. Reminding the patient to take antiretroviral medications on time

   D. The benefits of a support group

18. Amyotrophic lateral sclerosis (ALS) results in

   A. Acute episodes of weakness followed by long stretches of remission

   B. Changes in mentation

   C. Progressive weakness and atrophy of muscles

   D. Weakness of only the arms and legs

16. Answer is C

A. Incorrect: Chemotherapy and blood transfusions are not interchangeable treatments.

B. Incorrect: Chemotherapy can be very effective in treating many cancers.

C. **Correct:** Chemotherapy can be used in palliative care. For example, it can be used to decrease the size of the tumor, which will decrease pain.

D. Incorrect: Chemotherapy is not always expensive.

17. Answer is A

A. **Correct:** AIDS results in significant immunosuppression, which necessitates the need for the patient to be able to report any signs of infection.

B. Incorrect: Understanding universal precautions is important, but not what the nurse should begin with.

C. Incorrect: Though it is important for patients with HIV to take retroviral medications on a set schedule, it is HIV not AIDS that can be held in check with retroviral medications.

D. Incorrect: The patient may benefit from a support group, but teaching them about signs of infection takes precedence.

18. Answer is C

A. Incorrect: Remissions are not seen with ALS.

B. Incorrect: Usually there is no change in mentation.

C. **Correct:** ALS is a motor neuron disease in the cerebral cortex, brainstem, and spinal cord, which results in progressive weakness and atrophy of muscles.

D. Incorrect: Symptoms of ALS are not limited to the peripheral muscles.

19. When caring for a patient with advanced kidney disease, the nurse needs to remember that the most compelling psychosocial issue for a patient is

A. Whether or not to have surgery

B. How to function with nephrostomy tubes

C. Whether or not to continue with dialysis

D. How to handle family members' anxiety

20. A barrel chest is seen in a patient with which of the following diseases?

A. Chronic bronchitis

B. Emphysema

C. Lung cancer

D. Restrictive lung disease

Pain

21. When monitoring a patient in pain, the most appropriate piece of assessment data to obtain is

A. Site

B. Medication history

C. Character

D. Intensity

19. Answer is C

A. Incorrect: Surgery is not usually an option in advanced kidney disease.

B. Incorrect: Nephrostomy tubes are generally not used in advanced kidney disease.

C. **Correct:** Stopping dialysis will result in the death of the patient in a few days, thus making it a very difficult decision for patients and their families.

D. Incorrect: Assisting with a family member's anxiety is always important but is not usually the most compelling issue that the patient with end stage kidney disease is dealing with.

20. Answer is B

A. Incorrect: Chronic bronchitis symptoms usually include an overweight patient, cyanosis and breath that is wheezing.

B. **Correct:** A barrel chest is seen in patients with emphysema.

C. Incorrect: A barrel chest is not seen with lung cancer.

D. Incorrect: Restrictive lung disease results in loss of lung tissue which causes limited lung expansion.

Pain

21. Answer is D

A. Incorrect: Knowing the site is important, but not the most important thing to assess.

B. Incorrect: Medication history is important, but not the most important thing to assess.

C. Incorrect: The character of pain is important, but not the most important thing to assess.

D. **Correct:** Pain intensity directly correlates with interference with the patient's quality of life.

22. The **MOST** accurate judge of the intensity of the patient's pain is the

   A. Physician

   B. Patient

   C. Spouse/family member

   D. Nurse

23. The recommended route of administration of opioid analgesics for patients with prolonged cancer pain is

   A. Intravenous

   B. Intramuscular

   C. Oral

   D. Rectal

24. A patient's complaints of sharp, burning, or shooting pain is typically considered to be

   A. Visceral

   B. Somatic

   C. Neuropathic

   D. Chronic

22. Answer is B

A. Incorrect: The physician can contribute to the overall assessment of the patient's pain, but only the patient can rate his/her perceived/experience of pain intensity.

B. **Correct:** Pain is a highly subjective experience; pain is whatever the experiencing person says it is, existing whenever the person experiencing it says it does.

C. Incorrect: The spouse or family can contribute to the overall assessment of the patient's pain, but only the patient can rate his/her perceived/experience of pain intensity.

D. Incorrect: The nurse can contribute to the overall assessment of the patient's pain, but only the patient can rate his/her perceived/experience of pain intensity.

23. Answer is C

A. Incorrect: Intravenous route is typically used for resolving acute pain episodes.

B. Incorrect: The intramuscular route should be avoided whenever possible.

C. **Correct:** The oral route is the least invasive method supporting a greater degree of comfort for the patient and family caregivers.

D. Incorrect: The rectal route can be an acceptable alternative when the patient is no longer able to take meds orally.

24. Answer is C

A. Incorrect: Visceral pain is usually described as cramping, pressure and deep aches.

B. Incorrect: Somatic pain is usually associated with movement and described as deep, dull aches with easy point of origin by the patient.

C. **Correct:** Neuropathic pain is a result from actual injury to nerves, which typically represents itself with the classic signs of sharp shooting, burning descriptions by patients.

D. Incorrect: Chronic pain refers to the cyclical, ongoing occurrence of pain associated with chronic conditions.

25. Indicators of pain for a nonverbal patient in the final days of life include all of the following **EXCEPT**

A. Furrowed brow

B. Moaning

C. Guarding

D. Muscle relaxation

26. Evaluative data following oral administration of a short-acting analgesic (oxycodone) to a patient in pain should be assessed at

A. 30 minutes

B. 4 hours

C. 2 hours

D. End of shift

27. A dose of opioid that loses its effectiveness over time is called

A. Addiction

B. Analgesic ceiling

C. Physical dependence

D. Tolerance

25. Answer is D

A. Incorrect: A furrowed brow or facial grimacing may suggest the nonverbal patient is suffering in pain.

B. Incorrect: Moaning or vocalizations may suggest the nonverbal patient is suffering in pain.

C. Incorrect: Physical guarding with repositioning may suggest the nonverbal patient is suffering in pain.

D. **Correct:** Muscles are more likely to tense with pain.

26. Answer is A

A. **Correct:** Short-acting analgesics taken orally absorb into the body's circulation from the stomach and typically contribute effect within 30 minutes following administration.

B. Incorrect: Oxycodone has duration of action of 4–5 hours.

C. Incorrect: You need to know before 2 hours if the pain medication is not working.

D. Incorrect: Pain medication effectiveness is evaluated based on the onset of action and the time given, not when a shift ends or starts.

27. Answer is D

A. Incorrect: Addiction is an overwhelming involvement with obtaining and using a drug to its psychic effects.

B. Incorrect: Analgesic ceiling is a dose beyond which additional analgesic effect is not obtained.

C. Incorrect: Physical dependence occurs when after repeated administration of an opioid, withdrawal symptoms occur when the drug is not taken.

D. **Correct:** Tolerance occurs when after repeated administration of an opioid, a given dose begins to lose its effectiveness; first in duration of action; second in overall effectiveness. Dose should be gradually titrated upward to maintain the opioid's effectiveness.

28. Osteoarthritic pain is an example of which type of pain?

A. Referred

B. Somatic

C. Visceral

D. Neuropathic

29. Which of the following is an adverse effect of NSAIDs (nonsteroidal anti-inflammatory drugs)?

A. Hypersensitive hearing

B. Inhibition of platelet aggregation

C. Liver malfunction

D. Itching

30. When beginning a tricyclic antidepressant for the treatment of neuropathic pain, which of the following should be included in patient and family teaching?

A. Anticholinergic side effects may lead to diarrhea

B. Hyperactivity is a side effect

C. Hypertension may cause dizziness

D. Response may be delayed 3–7 days

28. Answer is B

A. Incorrect: Referred pain is felt at a site distant from the origin of the pain.

B. **Correct:** Somatic pain is a well-localized pain that can be musculoskeletal in nature.

C. Incorrect: Visceral pain is poorly localized and arises from organs.

D. Incorrect: Neuropathic pain results from actual injury to nerves rather than stimulation of nerve endings.

29. Answer is B

A. Incorrect: An adverse effect of NSAIDs is tinnitus and decreased hearing.

B. **Correct:** Inhibition of platelet aggregation is an adverse effect of NSAIDs.

C. Incorrect: Acetaminophen can have an adverse effect on the liver, not NSAIDs.

D. Incorrect: Itching is seen as a side effect of opioids, not NSAIDs.

30. Answer is D

A. Incorrect: The anticholinergic side effects of tricyclic antidepressants could lead to constipation.

B. Incorrect: Sedation is a side effect of tricyclic antidepressants.

C. Incorrect: Tricyclic antidepressants have a side effect of orthostatic hypotension, which could cause dizziness.

D. **Correct:** The response to tricyclic antidepressants may be delayed by 3–7 days after therapy is begun.

31. The son of a 72-year-old female in the middle stages of Alzheimer's disease reports that just since last night she has been very afraid that the IRS is going to arrest her. This behavior is most likely a result of

A. Aggression

B. Delirium

C. Confusion

D. Worsening of the Alzheimer's disease

32. Which of the following is **NOT** an etiology of agitation?

A. Brain tumor

B. Unrelieved pain

C. Noise

D. Metabolic disturbance

33. When working with a patient with agitation, patient and family education should include all of the following **EXCEPT**

A. Intermittent nature of most confusion

B. Safety needs

C. Compliance with bowel and bladder regimen

D. Food will make it worse

31. Answer is B

A. Incorrect: No reports of violent behavior were reported.

B. **Correct:** Exaggerated emotions like paranoia that develop over a short period of time are consistent with delirium.

C. Incorrect: The patient has become increasingly confused, but the paranoia would not be the result of just her confusion.

D. Incorrect: Alzheimer's disease is a slowly progressive disease. When changes occur over a short period, another cause must be looked into.

32. Answer is C

A. Incorrect: A brain tumor can cause agitation.

B. Incorrect: Unrelieved pain can cause agitation.

C. **Correct:** While noise *may* be a factor, it is not a true etiology. Need to assess for physiological and then psychological etiologies.

D. Incorrect: Metabolic disturbances can cause agitation.

33. Answer is D

A. Incorrect: It is important to teach patients and families that confusion, which can lead to agitation, is often intermittent.

B. Incorrect: It is very important to teach about safety issues when working with confused or agitated patients.

C. Incorrect: Bowel and bladder functioning is important for all patients, but especially so when working with a patient who may not be able to attend to their own needs. Constipation and urinary tract infections can make the agitations worse.

D. **Correct:** There are no foods that will make agitation worse, though feelings of hunger may.

34. Which of the following etiologies of ascites is **FALSE**?

A. Decreased plasma oncotic pressure

B. Lymphatic obstruction due to tumor infiltration

C. Portal hypertension

D. Portal hypotension

35. Ascites is the accumulation of?

A. Bile in the peritoneal cavity

B. Excessive fluid in the interstitial spaces of the abdomen

C. Excessive fluid in the peritoneal cavity

D. Fluid in the muscles of both the large and small intestines

36. Expected findings during an assessment of a patient with ascites would include

A. Dehydration

B. Increased bowel sounds

C. Hunger

D. Weight loss

34. Answer is D

A. Incorrect: Decreased plasma oncotic pressure can contribute to ascites.

B. Incorrect: Lymphatic obstruction due to tumor infiltration can contribute to ascites.

C. Incorrect: Portal hypertension can contribute to ascites.

D. **Correct:** Obstruction of portal vessels causing leakage, results in portal hyp**er**tension

35. Answer is C

A. Incorrect: Bile in the peritoneal cavity is not ascites.

B. Incorrect: Accumulation of fluid in interstitial spaces is edema.

C. **Correct:** Ascites is the accumulation of excessive amounts of fluid in the peritoneal cavity.

D. Incorrect: An accumulation of fluid in muscle tissue is edema.

36. Answer is A

A. **Correct:** Because so much fluid has been diverted to the abdominal cavity, dehydration is common in persons with ascites.

B. Incorrect: Bowel sounds may be decreased due to the pressure of the fluid on the bowels.

C. Incorrect: Anorexia or early satiety is common.

D. Incorrect: Weight gain is an expected finding with ascites.

37. Which of the following is **NOT** a likely etiology of a bowel obstruction?

A. Crohn's disease

B. Diuretics

C. External compression of the intestinal lumen

D. Gastric ulcer

38. When assessing a person with a bowel obstruction, it is important to assess for all of the following **EXCEPT**

A. Pain

B. Nausea and vomiting

C. Restless legs

D. Diarrhea

39. Seizures are

A. An increase in the pressure within the cranial cavity due to increased volume of fluid or mass

B. Intermittent tonic, clonic movements caused by a large number of neurons discharging abnormally

C. A sensation of numbness, prickling, or tingling; heightened sensitivity

D. Twitching or brief spasm of a muscle or muscle group

37. Answer is D

A. Incorrect: The inflammatory processes of Crohn's disease could cause a bowel obstruction.

B. Incorrect: Medications like diuretics that can cause hypokalemia can cause peristalsis to slow or stop.

C. Incorrect: External compression from a tumor or adhesions could cause a bowel obstruction.

D. **Correct:** A gastric ulcer in of itself would not cause a bowel obstruction.

38. Answer is C

A. Incorrect: Pain in a bowel obstruction is from the intestine's attempts to move the obstruction. It is also important to note if the pain decreases or goes away, as it could indicate worsening of the obstruction.

B. Incorrect: Nausea is frequently seen with a bowel obstruction. Vomiting occurs with a high obstruction as peristalsis may be reversed in an attempt to expel the obstruction. It is important to document the characteristic of the emesis.

C. **Correct:** Restless legs have nothing to do with bowel obstruction.

D. Incorrect: Diarrhea may occur due to overflow of feces around an incomplete obstruction or fecal impaction.

39. Answer is B

A. Incorrect: An increase in the pressure within the cranial activity due to increased volume of fluid or mass is increased intracranial pressure.

B. **Correct:** Intermittent tonic, clonic movements or convulsions caused by a large number of neurons discharging abnormally are seizures.

C. Incorrect: Paresthesia is a sensation of numbness, prickling, or tingling; heightened sensitivity.

D. Incorrect: Twitching or brief spasm of a muscle or muscle group is myoclonus.

40. Which of the following is **NOT** a possible etiology of seizures?

A. Brain tumor

B. Genetics

C. Infection

D. Stroke

Communication

41. Which of the following statements reflects poor or inappropriate active listening skills while interacting with a patient?

A. Adjusting your position to face the patient

B. Acknowledging what the person is telling you by nodding your head

C. Asking for clarification when necessary

D. Sitting with your arms crossed

42. You want to prepare the environment to facilitate a conversation with Mr. Gonzalez and his family. Which of the following actions is **MOST** appropriate?

A. Asking if it's okay to turn off the TV

B. Standing up so you can see everyone in the room

C. Ensuring that everyone has a beverage

D. Putting your cellular phone on the table so you can answer it quickly

40. Answer is B

A. Incorrect: Brain tumors can be a cause of seizures.

B. **Correct:** There is no research correlating genetics with seizures.

C. Incorrect: Infections can be a cause of seizures.

D. Incorrect: Cerebral vascular accidents or strokes can be causes of seizures.

Communication

41. Answer is D

A. Incorrect: Adjusting your position to face the patient reflects good active listening.

B. Incorrect: Acknowledging what the person is telling you by nodding your head reflects good active listening.

C. Incorrect: Asking for clarification when necessary reflects good active listening.

D. **Correct:** Sitting with your arms crossed is nonverbal communication that suggests you are not listening or are not open to what the person is saying.

42. Answer is A

A. **Correct:** Turning off the TV will remove distractions that make it difficult to focus on the conversation. However, you should ask permission from the family to turn the TV off.

B. Incorrect: Putting yourself "higher" than the person to whom you are speaking can cause the other person to feel less important or powerful.

C. Incorrect: Having something to drink is unlikely to make it easier to have a discussion with the patient and family.

D. Incorrect: Your cellular phone should be turned off during this time or placed on "mute."

43. Which of the following statements about silence in communication is **FALSE**? Silence

A. May mean that the person is thinking deeply about something

B. Is an ineffective communication tool

C. May mean that a person needs more time to consider an answer

D. Can be a way to "be present" to a dying person

44. Words such as "work" and "family" may have different meanings to different people. What is the best way to determine what a dying person is trying to convey?

A. Fill in the blanks in your mind with what you know about a person's culture

B. Ask family members what the word means to them

C. Ask the person what he or she means

D. Consult a "cultural guide" to give you input about what the words mean in their culture

45. Which of the following is an important message to communicate to dying patients and their families?

A. "I know how you are feeling."

B. "I accept you."

C. "We know what is best for you now."

D. "It is now time to give up aggressive therapies."

43. Answer is B

A. Incorrect: This is a true statement.

B. **Correct:** Silence can be an effective and the most appropriate communication tool at the end of life.

C. Incorrect: This is a true statement.

D. Incorrect: This is a true statement.

44. Answer is C

A. Incorrect: Never guess what a person means. You can easily guess incorrectly.

B. Incorrect: The family member may not understand why you are asking them for the meaning of a particular word.

C. **Correct:** Asking the person directly always is the best source of information because each individual is different.

D. Incorrect: Cultural guides are important sources of general information about a particular group. However, people within a specific cultural or religious group often have very different beliefs, practices, and language. Always ask the person first to be sure about the meaning of words.

45. Answer is B

A. Incorrect: Only the person experiencing the particular loss knows how he or she feels. This statement can be very insulting to the person.

B. **Correct:** Communicating your complete acceptance of the dying person and his family is one of the most therapeutic acts you can perform.

C. Incorrect: The patient and family decide what is best for them.

D. Incorrect: This is a decision made by the patient and/or family with input from the team regarding treatment options.

46. When is the best time to talk with dying people about their concerns?

A. When the person demonstrates they are ready to talk

B. Anytime that is convenient for you

C. In the morning after the person has had breakfast

D. After the person has been medicated

47. Which of the following is the best way to help maintain hope for a dying person and his/her family?

A. Assure them that everything will be okay

B. Avoid talking about death

C. Talk about your religious beliefs

D. Help them identify realistic goals

48. Which of the following statements about hope at the end of life is **TRUE**?

A. Hope may increase at the end of life

B. Hope is often focused on a person's achievements in the last months of life

C. Family relationships are always a source of hope

D. Hope is possible only if the person believes in an afterlife

46. Answer is A

A. **Correct:** Whenever possible, take the lead from the patient and family.

B. Incorrect: The patient and family should determine when it is the appropriate time to talk about their concerns.

C. Incorrect: A recent meal or particular time of day should not determine the timing of conversations; the patient's and family's interest and willingness to talk determines the proper timing.

D. Incorrect: A particular medication may assist the patient to focus on a conversation, for example, he may be more willing and able to talk following his pain medication because he is comfortable; however, you should watch for an indication from the patient that he wants to talk rather than relying on a specific event.

47. Answer is D

A. Incorrect: Providing false assurances will undermine their trust in you and can threaten hope.

B. Incorrect: Talking about death may increase, decrease, or have no affect on a person's hope; it depends on the person.

C. Incorrect: Do not discuss your religious beliefs with patients and families. Follow their lead in discussing spiritual issues and focus on their beliefs and values.

D. **Correct:** Helping patients and families establish achievable goals is important in maintaining their hope.

48. Answer is A

A. **Correct:** Studies show that dying people can experience high levels of hope and that hope may increase as death nears.

B. Incorrect: Hope often becomes refocused for people with life-threatening illnesses. Relationships and spirituality often become more important sources of hope than achievements.

C. Incorrect: Family relationships either can be a source or a threat to hope; it depends on the quality of the relationship.

D. Incorrect: Although people's belief in an afterlife can be a source of hope, hopefulness at the end of life does not depend on this belief.

49. Which of the following statements reflects the symbolic language that sometimes is used by the person who nearing death?

A. "I am in pain."

B. "I need to go to the train station."

C. "Why is God making me suffer?"

D. "I need to make funeral arrangements."

50. Which of the following is the most appropriate response when dealing with an angry family member or patient?

A. Remember that anger is a normal part of the grieving process

B. Stand close to the person so you can restrain them quickly if necessary

C. Do not let the person express his or her frustrations

D. Tell the person that you need to leave

Culture

51. Characteristics of culture are

A. Continuously evolving, is learned, and is shared by experience

B. A guide for behavior, a survival kit and based on phenotypic differences

C. A guide for human behavior, is learned, and is transmitted biologically

D. The sum of genotypic and phenotypic differences in a group

49. Answer is B

A. Incorrect: This statement indicates that the person is experiencing physical or psycho-spiritual distress. It is not an example of symbolic language.

B. **Correct:** Dying people sometimes use symbols to express their feelings or their understandings about their own living and dying. One example of symbolic language is when the dying person talks about going on a trip, which may indicate a person's awareness that he/she is dying.

C. Incorrect: This statement indicates spiritual distress, not symbolic language.

D. Incorrect: This statement indicates a person's actual, rather than symbolic, need to prepare for his/her death.

50. Answer is A

A. **Correct:** Anger may reflect unresolved grief.

B. Incorrect: When dealing with an angry person, it is best to maintain a safe distance. Standing too close may threaten the person and leave you open to physical injury if the person becomes violent.

C. Incorrect: Always let a person express his frustration, provided he is not verbally abusive.

D. Incorrect: Generally, it is best to stay with the angry person, unless you feel the situation is unsafe. If you need to leave, tell the person why you are leaving and when you will return.

Culture

51. Answer is A

A. **Correct:** Continuously evolving, is learned, and is shared by experience are characteristics of culture.

B. Incorrect: Culture may guide behavior, but is not considered a survival kit and is not based on the expression of genes or phenotype.

C. Incorrect: Culture may guide behavior and is learned, but it is not transmitted biologically.

D. Incorrect: Culture is not based on hereditary traits (genotype) or the expression of genes (phenotype).

52. Characteristics of groups and beliefs and values may be studied in courses and in the literature. Health professionals should recognize which of the following when working with clients

A. All group members follow a prescribed set of values according to their cultural traditions

B. Every group has definite values that group members would not violate

C. Norms for behavior are written and may be enforced in times of cultural change

D. Variations exist in all groups and the degree of acculturation may influence the extent to which beliefs and values of the culture are followed

53. The process where a cultural group becomes more similar to the dominant group and learns the language of the dominant group is called

A. Acculturation

B. Adaptation

C. Evolution

D. Assimilation

54. Which of the following best describes Euro-American cultural values?

A. Freedom, competition, and youth

B. Health, education, and valuing older adults

C. Independence, money, and regulation

D. Time, generosity, and socialized medicine

52. Answer is D

A. Incorrect: Not all members of a particular group follow the traditions in the same way as others in their culture. Some members of that group may not follow any of the traditions of the culture.

B. Incorrect: Individuals in a group are free to decide if they want to follow a value or not.

C. Incorrect: Culture is usually taught by the parents and is rarely written. Cultural norms for behavior influence laws, which are enforced.

D. **Correct:** Variations do exist in all groups and the degree of acculturation may influence the extent to which beliefs and values of the culture are followed.

53. Answer is A

A. **Correct:** Acculturation is the process where a cultural group becomes more similar to the dominant group and learns the language of the dominant group.

B. Incorrect: Adaptation is the process of adjusting to a new environment.

C. Incorrect: Evolution is the changing of genetic traits over time.

D. Incorrect: Assimilation is the incorporation of another group's beliefs into an individual's personal beliefs and values.

54. Answer is A

A. **Correct:** Freedom, competition, and youth are values of Euro-American culture.

B. Incorrect: Euro-American culture does not value older adults.

C. Incorrect: Euro-American culture prefers freedom over regulations.

D. Incorrect: Most Euro-American cultures have not valued socialized medicine.

55. Race has received considerable attention in the media and scientific literature. Current thinking about race includes that it is

   A. A useful concept for classifying people and describing ecological differences

   B. A useful concept for classifying people by biological and geographic differences

   C. The scientific merit of race is questionable, no single gene can explain race, and people are more similar than different

   D. Useful for genetic purposes, developing species taxonomy, and differentiating geographic regions

56. The definitions of ethnic group and ethnicity include all of the following aspects **EXCEPT**

   A. A collective similarity in ancestors, history, and/or language

   B. A sense of shared peoplehood

   C. Socially, politically, or culturally constructed groups

   D. Superiority of one's own ways

57. Fong's CONFHER model provides a framework for cultural assessment which includes gathering information about all of the following **EXCEPT**

   A. Sexual orientation

   B. Communication style

   C. Family relationships

   D. Religion

55. Answer is C

A. Incorrect: Race does not describe ecological differences.

B. Incorrect: As genetically all humans are 99.9% the same at the DNA level, race is not useful in classifying differences.

C. **Correct:** The concept of biological race is not consistent with scientific data and does not explain human variation.

D. Incorrect: All humans belong to the same species.

56. Answer is D

A. Incorrect: A collective similarity in ancestors, history, and/or language is a part of ethnicity.

B. Incorrect: Members of an ethnic group do have a sense of "shared peoplehood."

C. Incorrect: Aspects of ethnicity include socially, politically, or culturally constructed groups.

D. **Correct:** Superiority in one's own ways is not an aspect of ethnicity.

57. Answer is A

A. **Correct:** Fong's CONFHER model includes Communication, Orientation, Nutrition, Family relationships, Health and health beliefs, Education, and Religion.

B. Incorrect: See A

C. Incorrect: See A

D. Incorrect: See A

58. Ethnocentrism is based on an assumption of

    A. Favorable traits will be maintained

    B. Superiority of one's own view

    C. Measurement of average tendency

    D. Immersion in an ethnic culture

59. All cultures have a death system. The death system in the United States culture supports

    A. Openly discussing death and dying

    B. Increasing awareness of our mortality

    C. Keeping death at a distance and denying death

    D. Completing advance directives

60. Cultural assessment refers to appraisal of

    A. Cultural matrixes

    B. Individual, groups, and community beliefs and values

    C. Individual and family beliefs and values

    D. 12 cultural domains

58. Answer is B

A. Incorrect: Ethnocentrism is not connected to the maintaining of favorable traits.

B. **Correct:** Ethnocentrism is the tendency of people to believe that their ways of thinking, acting, and believing are the only right and proper ways.

C. Incorrect: Average tendency is not connected to ethnocentrism.

D. Incorrect: Immersion in an ethnic culture is a way of learning about a particular group's practices.

59. Answer is C

A. Incorrect: The American culture is generally not comfortable talking about death.

B. Incorrect: Americans do not like to think about their mortality.

C. **Correct:** Americans generally prefer to keep death at a distance and deny death.

D. Incorrect: Many Americans are reluctant to complete advance directives as it requires them to think about their death.

60. Answer is B

A. Incorrect: An appraisal of a cultural matrix would not give relevant assessment data.

B. **Correct:** A cultural assessment must include the individual, group, and their community.

C. Incorrect: The community must be included in a cultural assessment.

D. Incorrect: While there are models for cultural assessment that list domains, a cultural assessment is not limited to a certain list of things.

61. A 25-year-old Native American man asks the hospice nurse "What is really going on with my cancer? I don't think that my doctor is telling me the truth. She looks everywhere but at me when she talks to me." What has most likely happened that has made this patient feel that his doctor is not telling him the truth?

A. Because many Native Americans defer decision making to older family members, the doctor does not want to give too much information to the patient

B. The patient's cancer is of a type that giving a prognosis is extremely difficult

C. The doctor is shy

D. Because many Native Americans avoid eye contact, the doctor has assumed that this patient would not want to make eye contact

62. Culturally competent healthcare providers

A. Appreciate differences in people and are willing to learn

B. Have a desire to be culturally competent

C. Recognize building relationships takes time

D. All of the above

63. The United States is a multicultural society. According to the 2000 census the population group that has experienced the most growth is

A. Asian

B. Hispanic/Latino

C. American Indian

D. White

61. Answer is D

A. Incorrect: Some Native American tribes have large extended families that are involved in decision-making, but there is no indication that this is happening in this case.

B. Incorrect: If a patient has a cancer that is more difficult to determine a prognosis, the physician would include that with the information that they give to the patient.

C. Incorrect: While the doctor may be shy, she most likely is purposefully not making eye contact with the patient.

D. **Correct:** Many Native Americans do avoid eye contact, but it cannot be assumed that all Native Americans follow this practice. It is best to ask the patient what he prefers before assuming that a particular cultural practice is followed by that individual.

62. Answer is D

A. Incorrect: See D

B. Incorrect: See D

C. Incorrect: See D

D. **Correct:** Culturally competent healthcare providers appreciate differences in people and are willing to learn, have a desire to be culturally competent and recognize building relationships takes time.

63. Answer is B

A. Incorrect: The Asian population is growing, but not as much as the Hispanic/Latino population.

B. **Correct:** The Hispanic/Latino population has increased almost 58% in the past decade.

C. Incorrect: The Native American population is growing, but not as much as the Hispanic/Latino population.

D. Incorrect: The White population is shrinking.

Spirituality

64. During a dressing change, your patient asks "Why did I get cancer?" The best response would be

    A. Tell her that it was probably caused by her diet or lifestyle

    B. Tell her you will ask her doctor and get back to her with an answer later

    C. Explain that no one knows the true cause of cancer

    D. Encourage her to talk about her feelings related to her disease and be a good listener

65. Spirituality is

    A. The same as religion

    B. Only important to patients who believe in God

    C. Connection with self, neighbor, nature, God, or a higher being that moves one beyond oneself

    D. A and C

66. Religion is

    A. An organized effort to express one's spirituality

    B. A set of beliefs and behaviors

    C. Not the same as spirituality

    D. All of the above

Spirituality

64. Answer is D

A. Incorrect: No one knows for sure what causes cancer in an individual and such an answer would only make her feel guilty.

B. Incorrect: This is an evasive answer that does not address the patient's real concern. The doctor probably does not have an answer either.

C. Incorrect: While it is true that no one knows the true cause of cancer, the patient is asking a much deeper question and is trying to understand the meaning of her cancer and her life and death.

D. **Correct:** The patient needs to talk about her feelings and her own understanding of why she got ill and is dying. There is no right answer to her question. She is probably struggling to find some meaning in her life and some reason for her illness.

65. Answer is C

A. Incorrect: Religion is beliefs and practices used by some persons to express their spirituality.

B. Incorrect: A patient can be very spiritual and have strong beliefs without believing in God.

C. **Correct:** Spirituality refers to one's connection to any of these forces.

D. Incorrect: Only C is correct.

66. Answer is D

A. Incorrect: See D

B. Incorrect: See D

C. Incorrect: See D

D. **Correct:** Religion is all three (A, B, and C): an organized effort to express spirituality, a set of beliefs and behaviors and is not the same as spirituality.

67. Which of the following is **TRUE** about spiritual care in hospice? It

   A. Is only to be provided by the chaplain

   B. Does not affect how a person dies

   C. Includes all team members listening, accepting, and talking with patients and families about life and its meaning

   D. Is not a responsibility of the licensed practical/vocational nurse

68. Life review is

   A. An evaluation of the patient's health history

   B. That part of the team meeting when the social worker presents the patient's family history

   C. The patient's discussion of his or her life and its meaning

   D. Always the responsibility of the social worker

69. Roman Catholic beliefs and practices include all of the following **EXCEPT**

   A. Praying the rosary

   B. Receiving communion and the Sacrament of the Sick

   C. Observing Shiva

   D. Using symbols such as the cross or statues of saints

67. Answer is C

A. Incorrect: All team members have a role in the spiritual care of the hospice patient and family.

B. Incorrect: Spiritual care is usually very important to how a person dies.

C. **Correct:** All team members should be involved in communicating and accepting patient's and family's beliefs about life and its meaning.

D. Incorrect: The licensed practical/vocational nurse is responsible for responding to the spiritual needs of the patient and family.

68. Answer is C

A. Incorrect: Life review may include some health history, but the patient's health is not the primary focus.

B. Incorrect: Life review is something the patient (not a team member) does.

C. **Correct:** Life review is the patient's own review of his or her life and the meaning of that life.

D. Incorrect: All team members can be involved in a patient's life review.

69. Answer is C

A. Incorrect: Praying the rosary is a common Catholic practice.

B. Incorrect: Catholics may receive the Sacrament of the Sick when ill.

C. **Correct:** Observing Shiva is a Jewish practice.

D. Incorrect: Catholics often use symbols such as the cross or statues of saints to express or honor their faith.

70. Which of the following is a practice of a Muslim?

A. Cleaning the body before prayer

B. Reading from the Bible

C. Praying once daily at sunset

D. Burying the body within 24 hours of the death

71. Protestants believe

A. God speaks through the Bible

B. Believers go to heaven

C. Jesus' death provides salvation

D. All of the above

72. A licensed practical/vocational nurse should provide spiritual care because

A. Not all hospices can afford to hire a chaplain

B. The other team members are too busy

C. It does not require any special training or experience

D. Spiritual needs can come up at any time and the response should be immediate

70. Answer is A

A. **Correct:** Muslims always wash before prayer.

B. Incorrect: The Holy Book of the Muslim faith is the Quran.

C. Incorrect: Muslims pray five times daily.

D. Incorrect: Members of the Jewish faith bury the body within 24 hours of the death except when it falls on the Sabbath.

71. Answer is D

A. Incorrect: See D

B. Incorrect: See D

C. Incorrect: See D

D. **Correct:** Protestants believe all three: God speaks through the Bible, believers go to heaven, and Jesus' death provides salvation.

72. Answer is D

A. Incorrect: Most hospices do have chaplains available, but other team members must respond to spiritual needs as they arise.

B. Incorrect: Everyone on the team may be very busy, but everyone must take the time to respond to spiritual needs.

C. Incorrect: Providing spiritual care requires an understanding of the spiritual needs of the patient and family and the best way to respond.

D. **Correct:** Spiritual needs can come up at any time and every team member should be able to respond in a helpful manner.

73. If a patient has dementia, the licensed practical/vocational nurse should

A. Not upset the family by talking about the patient's past

B. Help the family remember and celebrate the patient's life before the disease

C. Be concerned with only the physical needs of the patient

D. Discourage family visits that might upset the patient

Pediatrics

74. According to Piaget, what is the primary stage of growth and development for children ages 3 to 7 years?

A. Concrete operational

B. Formal operational

C. Pre-operational

D. Sensory-motor

75. Grieving in a child begins

A. After the death of a loved one

B. Upon the realization that something is seriously wrong

C. When the child is involved in funeral rituals

D. When the child learns that someone is dying

73. Answer is B

A. Incorrect: Talking about the patient's past is usually helpful to the family as they remember their loved one as the person he or she was before the illness.

B. **Correct:** Talking about the life of the person who now has dementia helps the family remember the person they knew and loved before the illness.

C. Incorrect: Hospice and palliative care considers all aspects of the person—physical, emotional, social, and spiritual.

D. Incorrect: Family visits are helpful to the family and usually do not upset the patient.

Pediatrics

74. Answer is C

A. Incorrect: Concrete operational is the stage for 7- to 12-year-olds.

B. Incorrect: Formational operational is the stage for 12- to 18-year-olds.

C. **Correct:** Pre-operational is the stage for 3- to 7-year-olds. Current standards of care mandate that an understanding of the stages of development be interwoven into care for all individuals but most especially children so that care provided is done in a manner that is acceptable and understandable for the individual child.

D. Incorrect: Sensory motor is the stage for birth to 3 years of age.

75. Answer is B

A. Incorrect: See B

B. **Correct:** Grieving in a child begins upon the realization that something is seriously wrong or something has changed in the family.

C. Incorrect: The family may have the child involved in funeral rituals, but this is not when grieving begins.

D. Incorrect: See B

76. A child progresses to the next developmental stage based on

A. Age

B. Life experiences

C. Assessment tools

D. Physical development

77. Depression in the dying child

A. Is rare

B. Requires medications with a delayed onset

C. Should not be treated

D. Will have the same presentation as depression in the adult

76. Answer is B

A. Incorrect: Children of the same age can be at different stages.

B. **Correct:** All children/individuals must be assessed to determine at what stage of development they are and care planned appropriately. Although there are several theories on the stages of human development, they all agree that individuals move up and down these stages dependant on life circumstances. For example: a child that is potty trained will often regress to wetting themselves if a stressor is introduced into their lives such as a new sibling or separation from routine or primary caregivers. Appraisal of the child's developmental level is the first step toward a positive interaction, which reinforces the child's sense of security, mastery, and self-esteem. The nurse needs to be familiar with the child's developmental level to engage in any discussion on how they are physically feeling, for teaching related to care or disease progression, for selection of pain assessment tools and to determine method of any care to be provided.

C. Incorrect: Assessment tools cannot determine a child's developmental stage.

D. Incorrect: Physical development does not always coincide with developmental stage.

77. Answer is D

A. Incorrect: Depression in the dying child is not uncommon.

B. Incorrect: Depression in the dying child should be treated with immediate onset medications for a more rapid therapeutic effect.

C. Incorrect: Depression in the dying child should be treated.

D. **Correct:** Depression in the dying child will show the same symptoms as an adult.

78. The parents of a child who has been diagnosed with a terminal cancer asks you what they should say to their daughter. Which of the following is the best response to the parents' question?

A. "Children are children for such a little while we really need to protect them from the harsh realities of life especially if their diagnosis is terminal."

B. "She is probably aware that something is going on. Would you like to meet with the team so that they can help you decide what to tell her and how to talk to her?"

C. "You can tell her that she is sick and we will give her medicine to try to make her better."

D. "You should tell her that she has cancer using simple honest terms that you know she will understand."

79. An infant's fear of pain is related to

A. His/her understanding of pain

B. Inability to feel pain

C. Repeated painful experiences

D. Infants do not have the ability to fear pain

78. Answer is B

A. Incorrect: Recent research demonstrates that parents who avoid talking to their child about their illness and impending death often have much more difficult bereavements as well.

B. **Correct:** Discussion of treatment options and goals for care is essential. Discussion to clarify as much as possible, the intent, benefit, burden, and *meaning* of the treatments for all involved is critical to a comprehensive plan of care made in concert with the child, family, and healthcare providers. Upon discussion it may become evident that the understanding and perceptions of the goals of treatments may be shared, divergent, or conflicting among those involved and it is critical to reach a consensus for all concerned. It is our responsibility to clarify these issues with the primary caregivers of a child. Research has consistently shown that most children know that something is going on or that something is wrong and not communicating increases the sense of isolation and fear.

C. Incorrect: This statement would give the child incorrect information.

D. Incorrect: It is not our job however to take on the parental role and dismiss the parents' wishes or tell them what they should or should not say. It is our responsibility to honor the primary caregiver's wishes with the clear understanding that "we/healthcare providers" will not lie to a child when asked a direct question. Questions should be answered with simple, honest, and direct answers with respect and sensitivity to the primary caregiver's wishes.

79. Answer is C

A. Incorrect: In the first few months there is no apparent "understanding" of pain, but a baby does have a response to painful stimuli.

B. Incorrect: Infants do have the ability to feel pain.

C. **Correct:** After repeated painful experiences even the youngest infant learns to fear pain. Children develop anticipatory fear related to pain. It is important to explain all procedures/interactions that might be painful and to acknowledge the child's feelings.

D. Incorrect: Infants do have the ability to fear pain.

80. Which of the following is NOT true for pediatric hospice patients?

A. Children are not legally able to make decisions

B. Developmental levels/stages vary with each individual child/family

C. The ripple effect of a child's death is far greater than that of an adult

D. Reimbursement for pediatric care is the same as that for adult care

81. When managing pain in an infant, it is important to remember that

A. Adult doses can be cut in half for a child under the age of one year

B. Infants cannot effectively use as many drugs as adults can

C. The infant's nervous system is not developed enough to allow them to experience pain

D. What is painful for an adult is painful for an infant

80. Answer is D

A. Incorrect: Most children are unable to give legal consent regarding treatment, however determining assent vs. dissent is important. Children as young as 2 have been shown to be able to communicate likes vs. dislikes and children as young as 7 are considered old enough to give formal consent/dissent.

B. Incorrect: It is important to consider developmental stages as the context upon which to base explanations, education, needs assessment and relevant approaches. Having a basic understanding of normal growth and development is essential to appropriately formulate the plan of care for the individual child and family. Children have varied conceptions of and reactions to illness and death based on the following factors: age developmental level; family/religious/cultural norms; cognitive, intellectual and emotional maturity in order to plan care, teaching and basic communication in the best way possible.

C. Incorrect: In the "natural" order individuals die of old age. However, when a child dies the ripple effect extends far beyond the immediate circle of family and friends, encompassing school, church community, residential neighborhood, sports community, etc.

D. **Correct:** Traditional hospice care in the United States was designed for the care of dying adults, it is regulated by Medicare and has guidelines and regulations many parents and healthcare providers find impossible to accept. Less than 20% of children eligible for hospice care actually enroll in a hospice program.

81. Answer is D

A. Incorrect: This is not a correct statement. Infant and children's medication dosage must be carefully calculated according to weight by the registered nurse with the physician and pharmacist using established resources.

B. Incorrect: Children and infants can use many of the same medications that adults use. The registered nurse will work with the physician and pharmacist to determine the best medications for each child.

C. Incorrect: An infant is able to feel pain.

D. **Correct:** The Golden Rule of pain management in children is "what is painful for an adult is painful to a child or infant."

82. Which of the following is a common need of children facing death?

    A. Keep information to a minimum

    B. Downplaying fears and anxieties

    C. Do care activities for them

    D. Continued routine activities

83. At what age does stranger anxiety usually occur?

    A. 3 to 12 months

    B. 7 months to 3 years

    C. 18 months to 4 years

    D. 2 years to 4 years

82. Answer is D

A. Incorrect: Children need to have information about their condition.

B. Incorrect: Children will have questions, fears, anxieties, and need reassurance and support. Everyone needs someone that listens to them and children as well as adults need help with overwhelming feelings.

C. Incorrect: Involving the child and including them in their own care gives validation.

D. **Correct:** Normalization in the midst of extreme circumstances helps many face what the future holds. Focusing on living gives all a sense of control.

83. Answer is B

A. Incorrect: See B

B. **Correct:** Stranger anxiety typically occurs between 7 months to 3 years when it starts to decrease. Approach the infant/child in an unhurried manner to avoid frightening the infant/child. When frightened, the child may not allow interactions and you may not be able to perform your duties, causing undue stress to the infant/child/parents and yourself. Initial contact is best with parent holding baby or within close view; smile; approach should be unhurried and gentle, use soft voice, but not "baby" talk; avoid abrupt jerky movements and loud noises that may startle the child.

C. Incorrect: See B

D. Incorrect: See B

Family Caregivers

84. Recognizing the roles/needs of family caregivers involves which of the following?

    A. Preparing for impending death

    B. Looking at the developmental stage of the family

    C. Helping to reduce physical and emotional burden

    D. All of the above

85. Which of the following statements is a caregiver concern?

    A. Providing symptom management

    B. Their own physical health

    C. Administering medications

    D. All of the above

86. Interventions to help family caregivers with physical care should include providing

    A. Medical advice

    B. Psychological counseling

    C. Resources to help with physical care (i.e., nursing assistant)

    D. Financial counseling

Family Caregivers

84. Answer is D

   A. Incorrect: See D

   B. Incorrect: See D

   C. Incorrect: See D

   D. **Correct:** Family caregivers need to know what to look for as the patient's disease progresses such as signs and symptoms. Knowing the developmental stage of the family will help you know what kind of resources to provide regarding help with the patient and help for the family caregiver to reduce physical and emotional burdens.

85. Answer is D

   A. Incorrect: See D

   B. Incorrect: See D

   C. Incorrect: See D

   D. **Correct:** All of the statements are concerns for the family caregiver. As the disease gets worse, the patient's symptoms may get worse and additional symptoms may occur. A concern of the family caregiver is that they will not know what to do. Along with the physical symptoms, there is usually a need for the family caregiver to provide medications, especially pain meds and this can at first be very overwhelming. Many family caregivers battle their own health problems and even those who are healthy get very tired and need a rest. These are important concerns to be addressed by the nurse and reinforced by other members of the healthcare team.

86. Answer is C

   A. Incorrect: Medical advice is the domain of the physician and appropriate nursing personnel.

   B. Incorrect: Psychological counseling should be provided by trained personnel only.

   C. **Correct:** Your job is to provide resources to help with the physical care.

   D. Incorrect: Financial counseling should be provided by trained personnel only.

87. Which of the following are emotional needs of family caregivers?

A. Coping skills and emotional validation

B. Counseling

C. Desire to let someone else take over

D. Need to distance themselves

88. Which emotions are **NOT** normal for family caregivers?

A. Anger

B. Helplessness

C. Suicidal thoughts

D. Fear

89. Why is the developmental stage of the family important to consider when planning care?

A. Families of elder patients will need less preparation for the death

B. The developmental stage will determine the care that the family needs

C. The illness affects the whole family

D. The younger the family, the more the death has an impact on the family

87. Answer is A

A. **Correct:** Most family caregivers want to help but they just feel inadequate. Most have not had prior experience. Providing them with skills to help them cope in identified areas needing help is invaluable. Because of feelings of inadequacy, providing emotional validation is like water in the desert.

B. Incorrect: Counseling is not always indicated.

C. Incorrect: Family caregivers want to stay in control.

D. Incorrect: Family caregivers do not like to feel unconnected.

88. Answer is C

A. Incorrect: Anger is a common feeling when a loved one is dying.

B. Incorrect: Helplessness is a common feeling when a loved one is dying.

C. **Correct:** Family caregivers will experience an array of emotions, even ones that may "wish this was all over and I know that sounds horrible." That is a fairly common statement when the disease process is prolonged. However, suicidal thoughts of any kind are not normal and should be reported immediately to the registered nurse and other appropriate personnel.

D. Incorrect: Fear is a common feeling when a loved one is dying.

89. Answer is C

A. Incorrect: Preparation for the death of an older person differs, but they do not need less.

B. Incorrect: The developmental stage of the family will guide care, but does not determine it as all families are different.

C. **Correct:** The developmental stage of the family is very important. Younger children will be affected differently than older children who will be affected differently than the spouse. If the family is in child bearing years, this will have a profound affect on a parent if it is a child who dies and likewise on the children if a parent dies. This is very different to an elderly person who loses a spouse of 50 years.

D. Incorrect: No one stage is impacted by death more or less than another stage.

90. Perceived lack of support from family and friends differs from actual lack of support in that perceived lack of support

A. Does not result in loneliness and isolation

B. Is not as authentic or as important

C. Is not different from actual lack of support

D. It can be assumed that it is the result of conflict within the family

91. Which intervention does **NOT** reflect the licensed practical/vocational nurse's role?

A. Addressing personal concerns of the family

B. Validating caregiver feelings

C. Offering to visit on off duty hours

D. Suggesting the help of a hospice volunteer

92. The main difference between religiosity and spirituality is

A. There is no real main difference

B. Religion is only concerned with rituals

C. Spirituality is only concerned with the soul

D. Religion is usually defined as a system of faith and worship, whereas spirituality is defined as connection with God or higher power

90. Answer is C

A. Incorrect: Both perceived and actual lack of support result in feelings of loneliness and isolation.

B. Incorrect: Perceived lack of support is as authentic and important as actual lack of support.

C. **Correct:** Think about a time when you *thought* you lost something or someone you loved. Those emotions were very real. It is the same with FAMILY CAREGIVERS who perceive a lack of support; the response is the same. The best thing to do is to inquire more about their feelings to possibly obtain information that would enable you or someone else to help them. Remember that emotions are neither right nor wrong, they just are. All behavior has meaning.

D. Incorrect: While both perceived and actual lack of support can be the result of family conflict, there are many possible reasons.

91. Answer is C

A. Incorrect: This is a role of the licensed practical/vocational nurse.

B. Incorrect: This is a role of the licensed practical/vocational nurse.

C. **Correct:** It is not the licensed practical/vocational nurse's role or duty to make visits on off duty hours.

D. Incorrect: This is a role of the licensed practical/vocational nurse.

92. Answer is D

A. Incorrect: There is a difference between religiosity and spirituality.

B. Incorrect: Rituals are only a part of religiosity.

C. Incorrect: Concern for the soul is only a part of spirituality.

D. **Correct:** This statement best reflects the differences between religiosity and spirituality.

93. Which of the following statements is **NOT** true regarding family caregivers?

A. Hope is not linked to a sense of purpose

B. Uncertainty is a common fear of family caregivers

C. Some family caregivers need rituals or sacraments to feel close to God

D. Finding meaning in the loved one's illness is important to the family caregiver

Bereavement

94. Which of the following is the correct definition of bereavement?

A. A strong need to remain close to, or to return to another individual

B. The outward signs of grief; the process one goes through adapting to a loss

C. Complex series of reactions following death, including grief and mourning

D. Intense, emotional loss caused by suffering

95. Parkes's tasks of grief are

A. Accept, experience, adjust, reinvest

B. Alarm, searching, mitigation, anger, new identity

C. Denial, anger, bargaining, depression, acceptance

D. Numbing, searching, disorganization, reorganization

93. Answer is A

A. **Correct:** Hope is linked to a sense of purpose.

B. Incorrect: Uncertainty is a common fear of family caregivers.

C. Incorrect: Rituals or sacraments are needed by some to feel closer to God.

D. Incorrect: Many family caregivers search for meaning in a loved one's illness.

Bereavement

94. Answer is C

A. Incorrect: Loss can result in the need to be closer to others, but this is not a definition of bereavement.

B. Incorrect: Adapting to a loss is only one aspect of bereavement.

C. **Correct:** Bereavement incorporates grief and mourning.

D. Incorrect: Bereavement includes losses of any kind.

95. Answer is B

A. Incorrect: Accept the reality of the loss, experience the pain or grief, adjust to an environment without the deceased and withdraw emotional energy and reinvest in another relationship are Worden's Tasks.

B. **Correct:** Alarm, searching, mitigation, anger, and gaining new identity are Parkes's tasks of grief.

C. Incorrect: Denial, anger, bargaining, depression, and acceptance are Kübler-Ross's stages of grief.

D. Incorrect: Numbing with possible anguish and anger, searching and longing, disorganization and despair, and reorganization are Bowlby's tasks of grief.

96. Which of the following is an example of age and demographics making a difference in the way people experience bereavement?

    A. Cultural differences should not affect end-of-life care

    B. Men are more inclined to seek help

    C. Older adults do not consider death to be a part of normal aging

    D. Older children's bereavement can be complicated by failure in communication

97. Which statement best reflects an effective assessment during a time of grieving?

    A. Grieving is not integrated into the conversation

    B. Answers to assessment questions are not to be used for other purposes

    C. Only includes verbal responses

    D. Includes nurturance, comfort, touch, sense of presence, and compassion

98. Those at risk for complicated grief include which of the following?

    A. Traumatic death

    B. Death of a child

    C. Those having a low self image

    D. All of the above

96. Answer is D

A. Incorrect: Cultural differences do affect end of life.

B. Incorrect: Men and women experience loss differently. Women generally are more emotional and need to talk, whereas men tend to hold in their emotions and keep to themselves. Though women are more likely to seek help, each person must be treated as an individual.

C. Incorrect: Many older adults do consider death to be a normal part of aging.

D. **Correct:** Due to the emotional and maturational stages of life, children will experience and respond to loss much differently than adults. An older child's bereavement can be complicated by failures in communication.

97. Answer is D

A. Incorrect: A good assessment is not just limited to the obvious or to a check-off list.

B. Incorrect: Needs identified during an assessment are used to guide the plan of care.

C. Incorrect: Non-verbal responses including body language and expressions are as equally important as verbal responses.

D. **Correct:** A good assessment provides a sense of caring about the patient as a person and not just a disease.

98. Answer is D

A. Incorrect: See D

B. Incorrect: See D

C. Incorrect: See D

D. **Correct:** The list is too long to discuss each risk however; the complications arise from unresolved issues and emotions in a person's life that are triggered by the patient's death.

99. Examples of complicated grief include all of the following **EXCEPT**

A. Exaggerated grief

B. Depression

C. Absent grief

D. Doing something fun

100. Which of the following statements about having unusual experiences, such as seeing a family member who had died, is **NOT** true?

A. Often discounted as dreams or hallucinations

B. Viewed as common

C. Can have a therapeutic effect

D. Provides a sense of the loved one being okay

101. Which of the following statements is **TRUE** regarding grief in nurses?

A. Grief over a close patient relationship may result in a culmination of grief experienced from many deaths

B. Nurses build up an "immunity" to grief

C. Relationships with patients that were not close to the nurse are not mourned

D. Whether the nurse considers the death a "good" or "bad" death does not effect their grieving

99. Answer is D

A. Incorrect: Exaggerated grief is an example of complicated grief.

B. Incorrect: Depression is an example of complicated grief.

C. Incorrect: Absent grief is an example of complicated grief.

D. **Correct:** Doing something fun is a sign of healthy grief, not complicated grief.

100. Answer is B

A. Incorrect: Unusual experiences are often discounted as dreams or hallucinations.

B. **Correct:** Having an unusual experience is NOT common, hence why patients are slow to share the experience and others tend to assign a physical reason for it.

C. Incorrect: Unusual experiences can have a therapeutic effect.

D. Incorrect: Unusual experiences can provide a sense of the loved one being okay.

101. Answer is A

A. **Correct:** Nurses usually do not have time, or enough time to grieve adequately when a patient dies due to job responsibilities including other patients. So when a patient with whom the nurse has been close dies, there can be an accumulated emotional response that occurs from "stuffing emotions."

B. Incorrect: Nurses may become callous, but they are not immune to grief.

C. Incorrect: The loss is mourned regardless of the type of relationship experienced.

D. Incorrect: Nurses cope better with what they consider to have been a good death.

102. Which statement reflects the best way to help staff cope with grief at work?

A. Write a letter to your supervisor

B. Initiate action on an individual, managerial, and institutional level

C. Refuse to take care of imminently dying patients

D. Staff meeting

103. Which statement is **NOT** true about bereavement?

A. Bereavement is changing and dynamic

B. There is a need for spiritual support

C. Provides nurses with opportunities to help through listening, communicating, teaching, or facilitating support groups

D. Only begins after death

Care at the Time of Dying

104. "Role-modeling" patient care for family members of a patient with dementia is best characterized by the nurse

A. Addressing the patient by name every time she/he enters the room

B. Asking a family member to repeat care instructions

C. Determining learning barriers the patient may have

D. Referring a chaplain in response to the request for a religious ritual

102. Answer is B

A. Incorrect: Writing a letter to your supervisor may or may not help; it depends on the supervisor.

B. **Correct:** Initiating action on an individual, managerial, and institutional level would allow several means by which staff could choose to help them cope with grief.

C. Incorrect: Refusing to take care of dying patients is not learning to cope with grief; it is denying that it happens. You as a nurse will not grow professionally or personally by taking this action.

D. Incorrect: Not everyone may feel comfortable sharing in a group such as a staff meeting.

103. Answer is D

A. Incorrect: Bereavement does not only begin after death. It can occur throughout the whole loss process. Bereavement is changing and dynamic and is not linear.

B. Incorrect: Spiritual support is very much needed and is a prime opportunity for nurses to serve compassion and kindness to the family members.

C. Incorrect: Bereavement does provide nurses with opportunities to help through listening, communicating, teaching, or facilitating support groups.

D. **Correct:** The bereavement process begins before death.

Care at the Time of Dying

104. Answer is A

A. **Correct:** This is the only example of demonstrating appropriate patient care that family members can adopt.

B. Incorrect: A good intervention, but not an example of role-modeling.

C. Incorrect: A good intervention, but not an example of role-modeling.

D. Incorrect: A good intervention, but not an example of role-modeling.

105. Which of the following is most likely to be burdensome to the patient during the dying phase?

A. A culturally sensitive approach

B. Frequent staff presence

C. Routine vital signs

D. Symptom relief

106. In a situation where the patient and a family member express a difference of opinion about goals of care, which of the following is the most important guide for the healthcare team? The

A. Attending physician's recommendations

B. Nursing care plan

C. Opinion of the next-of-kin

D. Patient's preferences

107. A patient's husband reports to you his concern that his dying wife is having trouble breathing. You observe that the patient has started a Cheyne-Stokes breathing pattern. Your best response to the patient's husband is

A. "This breathing pattern is caused by your wife's pain medication."

B. "Your wife may need oxygen to make her more comfortable."

C. "We will contact the doctor for some medication for this problem."

D. "This is an expected part of the dying process."

105. Answer is C

A. Incorrect: A culturally sensitive approach to care is not burdensome by definition.

B. Incorrect: Frequent staff presence could be burdensome if disruptive, but is a recommended intervention, as staff tend to spend too little, rather than too much time with dying patients in many settings.

C. **Correct:** Routine vital signs, especially BP and temperature are often burdensome to actively dying patients especially for patients who are confused, delirious, or have unmanaged pain or nausea.

D. Incorrect: Symptom relief is not burdensome by definition.

106. Answer is D

A. Incorrect: Patient preferences, whether currently or previously expressed or documented, should always be the guide for end stage care over the opinions or recommendations of professional caregivers.

B. Incorrect: The nursing care plan should reflect the patient's preferences, but there is no guarantee that this occurs in all care settings.

C. Incorrect: The opinions and/or preferences of the patient's next of kin should only be considered if the patient cannot currently express preferences and they are not previously known, and there is no designated power of attorney for health affairs.

D. **Correct:** Patient preferences, whether currently or previously expressed or documented, should always be the guide for end stage care.

107. Answer is D

A. Incorrect: Cheyne-Stokes breathing is not caused by medications.

B. Incorrect: Oxygen therapy does not usually help dyspnea like Cheyne-Stokes breathing at the end of life.

C. Incorrect: Cheyne-Stokes is not distressful to the patient and therefore does not require any intervention, other than monitoring and family education and support.

D. **Correct:** Cheyne-Stokes is an expected part of the dying process.

108. Which of the following is the best example individualizing the care environment on an inpatient unit for a dying person?

A. Adhering to a consistent care routine

B. Asking the patient when he would like his food tray delivered

C. Ensuring a calm environment by closing the window blinds and door

D. Limiting the number of visitors during the night

109. You are caring for a patient who is alert and has his symptoms well-managed. However, his attending physician says this patient has very little time left to live. Which of the following spiritual interventions would be a priority? Ensuring that the

A. Chaplain provides counseling to this patient

B. Family's religious traditions are followed

C. Patient's existential concerns are addressed

D. Staff understand the teachings of the patient's religion

110. A patient with chronic pain tells you the pain does not seem as bad when he is playing his favorite card game. This could be considered a

A. Non-drug pain intervention

B. Patient who has a low level of pain

C. Reason to consider lowering the patient's pain medication

D. Cultural response to pain

108. Answer is B

A. Incorrect: A consistent care routine may be burdensome to the patient if it interferes with his/her comfort and rest.

B. **Correct:** This is the only answer where the patient's individual preference is elicited.

C. Incorrect: A calm environment may not be the correct intervention for a patient who needs distraction, is frightened of being alone, or if the quiet increases anxiety.

D. Incorrect: The patient may want many visitors at night, or on some nights.

109. Answer is C

A. Incorrect: Although chaplain assessment is almost always helpful, an individual chaplain may not be the best person to provide the actual counseling, as some patients would prefer another member of the healthcare team or their community religious/spiritual advisor to provide counseling.

B. Incorrect: The patient may not be concerned that his family or his own religious traditions are followed.

C. **Correct:** The patient's concerns are always priority.

D. Incorrect: Staff understanding of the teachings of the patient's religion may be helpful, but the patient may not follow all or most of his religion's teaching, or may have rejected some or all of it.

110. Answer is A

A. **Correct:** This is an example of distraction, a non-drug pain intervention.

B. Incorrect: The level of pain could not have been determined by the above information.

C. Incorrect: This would not be a reason to lower pain medication, as the patient is indicating he still has some pain and the distraction and pain medication may be a helpful combination for pain management.

D. Incorrect: This example of distraction has nothing to do with the patient's cultural background.

111. While bathing a patient with end stage cancer, you notice that both lower legs are cool to the touch, with areas of blue and purple coloring. This patient could most benefit from

A. A blood flow scan

B. Warm blankets to the legs

C. An increase in the rate of his oxygen therapy

D. A physical therapy consult

112. For a patient who is unable to communicate verbally, the most reliable sign that he or she may be in pain is

A. Furrowing of the brow

B. Picking at the bedclothes

C. General restlessness

D. Moaning with exhalation

113. Which of the following is most likely to assist with the grieving of family members at the time of death?

A. Limiting family members' time with the patient's body immediately after death

B. Ensuring that a staff member remains with the family at the patient's bedside at all times

C. Initiating prayers immediately after death, if the family is too distraught to do so

D. Facilitating family member participation in post-mortem care

111. Answer is B

A. Incorrect: This is a description of mottling, due to decreased circulation in the very last stages of dying. There is no effective intervention to reverse this process, so a blood flow scan would not be appropriate.

B. **Correct:** Warm blankets may provide symptom relief to those patients who also feel cold, as part of the decreased blood perfusion in the late dying stage.

C. Incorrect: Oxygen therapy has not been shown to reverse this process.

D. Incorrect: A physical therapy consult would be ineffective, as often these patients are hours to days from dying, once their skin begins mottling.

112. Answer is A

A. **Correct:** Furrowing of the brow is considered to be the most reliable nonverbal sign of pain.

B. Incorrect: Picking at bedclothes is a sign of delirium or other neurological dysfunction in the late dying phase.

C. Incorrect: General restlessness does indicate discomfort, but is more often due to urinary retention or constipation than pain.

D. Incorrect: If a patient moans when moved, that may or may not indicate pain. However, moaning with each exhalation is due to a relaxation of the throat muscles and can best be eliminated in some patients by repositioning.

113. Answer is D

A. Incorrect: It is not correct to limit family member time at the bedside immediately after death, but rather spending time with the body should be encouraged for those who wish to do so.

B. Incorrect: Facilitating family member participation means that families are given a choice if and how they may wish to participate in post-mortem care.

C. Incorrect: It should not be assumed that initiating prayers is appropriate. This should only be done as the family's request or with their permission.

D. **Correct:** This choice is critical in some cultures and with some relationships such as the death of a child.

Professionalism

114. Physical distress and fatigue are manifestations of

    A. Anorexia

    B. Stress

    C. Professionalism

    D. Relationships

115. Maintaining professional boundaries means to

    A. Limit interactions with others

    B. Foster dependence of patients and families

    C. Understand team member roles

    D. Explain to others what their role should be

116. Precepting new students is also called

    A. Advocacy

    B. Networking

    C. Peer review

    D. Mentoring

Professionalism

114. Answer is B

   A. Incorrect: Anorexia is having little or no appetite.

   B. **Correct:** Stress can be manifested by physical distress and fatigue.

   C. Incorrect: Professionalism is represented by the following characteristics: altruism, integrity, caring/compassion/communication, respect, responsibility/accountability, excellence/scholarship, and leadership.

   D. Incorrect: Relationships occur when people participate in communications.

115. Answer is C

   A. Incorrect: Professional boundaries should not limit interactions with others.

   B. Incorrect: Professional nurses should never be dependent on patients and families.

   C. **Correct:** It is imperative to understanding the roles of other team members in order to not overstep professional boundaries.

   D. Incorrect: The explanation of roles should be done by supervisors.

116. Answer is D

   A. Incorrect: Advocacy is the process and act of representing the wishes, values, or concerns of another individual who may be less able to do so.

   B. Incorrect: Networking is the communication with other hospice and palliative team members.

   C. Incorrect: Peer review is the evaluation of a colleague's work performance.

   D. **Correct:** Mentoring is sharing experiences and providing support and friendship in the workplace.

117. Participating in membership organizations is a part of

A. Professionalism

B. Licensure

C. Certification

D. Job requirements

118. PDCA stands for

A. Professionalism, dedication, certification, and advocacy

B. Professionalism, do, check, and act

C. Plan, do, check, and advocate

D. Plan, do, check, and act

119. The process and act of representing the wishes, values, or concerns of another individual who may be less able to do so is

A. Collaboration

B. Professionalism

C. Empathy

D. Advocacy

117. Answer is A

A. **Correct:** Professionalism is represented by the following characteristics: altruism, integrity, caring/compassion/communication, respect, responsibility/accountability, excellence/scholarship, and leadership.

B. Incorrect: Licensure is required by law to practice nursing.

C. Incorrect: Certification is a means of promoting professional development.

D. Incorrect: Job requirements are stipulations set by the employer for employment.

118. Answer is D

A. Incorrect: See D

B. Incorrect: See D

C. Incorrect: See D

D. **Correct:** Plan, do, check, and act are the four steps in an example of a quality improvement model.

119. Answer is D

A. Incorrect: Collaboration is working together with other individuals in a positive and effective manner where the combination of the knowledge and gifts of each individual in the group results in better outcomes for the patient and family.

B. Incorrect: Professionalism is represented by the following characteristics: altruism, integrity, caring/compassion/communication, respect, responsibility/accountability, excellence/scholarship, and leadership.

C. Incorrect: Empathy is demonstrating compassion.

D. **Correct:** This is the definition of advocacy.

120. Certified licensed practical/vocational hospice and palliative nurses use the following credentials

A. CHPLPN

B. CHPN

C. CHPLN

D. CHPNA

121. Professional growth and development includes all of the following **EXCEPT**

A. Participating in peer review

B. Providing self-care

C. Maintaining professional boundaries

D. Using the PDCA Cycle

122. Demonstrating knowledge, attitudes, behaviors, and skills consistent with the scope of practice is the definition of

A. Certification

B. Competency

C. Professionalism

D. Mentoring

120. Answer is C

A. Incorrect: CHPLPN is not an abbreviation for a hospice and palliative certification.

B. Incorrect: CHPN stands for Certified Hospice and Palliative Nurse.

C. **Correct:** CHPLN stands for Certified Hospice and Palliative Licensed Nurse.

D. Incorrect: CHPNA stands for Certified Hospice and Palliative Nursing Assistant.

121. Answer is D

A. Incorrect: Participating in peer review is a part of professional growth and development.

B. Incorrect: Providing self-care is part of professional growth and development.

C. Incorrect: Maintaining professional boundaries is a part of professional development.

D. **Correct:** The PDCA Cycle is a method of quality improvement.

122. Answer is C

A. Incorrect: Certification is a means of promoting professional development.

B. Incorrect: Competency is maintaining one's ability to be a nurse.

C. **Correct:** These are all part of being a professional.

D. Incorrect: Mentoring is sharing experiences and providing support and friendship in the work place.

123. A distinct body of knowledge that directs the licensed practical/vocational nurse in providing excellent care is the

A. PDCA Cycle

B. Boundaries of Professionalism

C. Scope of Practice

D. Standards of Care

124. Professional responsibilities include

A. Competency, advocacy, and mentoring

B. Networking, competency, and certification

C. Role-modeling, advocacy, and certification

D. Mentoring, advocacy, and being willing to cross boundaries

123. Answer is C

A. Incorrect: PDCA Cycle is a process of quality improvement.

B. Incorrect: Boundaries of professionalism are ground rules for professional behaviors.

C. **Correct:** Scope of practice is the activities the licensed practical/vocational nurse is legally permitted to perform as determined by their state board of nursing.

D. Incorrect: Standards of care identify the responsibilities for which licensed practical/vocational nurses, are accountable.

124. Answer is A

A. **Correct:** Competency, advocacy, and mentoring are all included in professional responsibilities.

B. Incorrect: While networking and certification are important to the professional nurse, they are not considered to be professional responsibilities.

C. Incorrect: Role-modeling and certification are important to the professional nurse, they are not considered to be professional responsibilities.

D. Incorrect: Being willing to cross boundaries is not a professional behavior or responsibility.

Case Studies and Answers

Case Studies for Discussion

Interdisciplinary Team

Case Study #1

Your Hospice Team has undergone some recent changes in personnel. In the past the IDT has appeared to function well in the allotted time. A new medical director has started. She is an oncologist who has been part of a multi-disciplinary cancer care team in a local hospital before starting with your hospice. This is her first job with a hospice. In addition, the patient care coordinator, who normally leads the IDT, is now on maternity leave. The hospice administrator has agreed to step in as leader of the weekly IDT. He has not attended an IDT in several weeks prior to the coordinator leaving, due to many administrative responsibilities.

At the medical director's first meeting, she directs her questions to the registered nurses about patient problems. She also spends significant time discussing anatomy and physiology of the patient's symptoms. The social workers and home health aides have not spoken. Some of them appear bored and start doing their paperwork in the meeting. The registered nurses and licensed practical/vocational nurses are asked many questions about the pathophysiology of symptoms. This is making some of the nurses anxious. The hospice administrator seems very interested in issues being discussed by the physician.

1. What are the signs that the team functioning is being compromised?

2. What factors may have contributed to the change in this team's functioning?

3. What barriers are present to effective interdisciplinary collaboration?

4. How would a well-functioning interdisciplinary team address this change in team dynamics and functioning?

Case Study #1 Answers

1. **Answer:** Only the nurses are being asked questions. It sounds like team members do not feel comfortable to bring up patient issues. The new leader is not demonstrating awareness of problems. The physician appears to be running the meeting, which is a major change from the previous role of medical director.

2. **Answer:** The hospice administrator may be unfamiliar with how the team functioned in the past. The new medical director may be thinking that the hospital or medical model she previously used is effective in the hospice setting. She may also be unsure of her role and wants to establish her credibility to this new group by addressing topics she is most comfortable with (i.e., disease states, anatomy, physiology).

3. **Answer:** Team members are not comfortable with questioning the new format, social workers and home health aides may feel left out, the physician and administrator are authority figures that members may feel uncertain about questioning.

4. **Answer:** Team members could bring up tactfully that this is a change in team function and want to discuss ways to achieve goals of the IDT. The leader could point out that social workers and home health aides need to bring up their concerns about the patients discussed. The medical director could acknowledge being new and not totally sure of her role and request feedback after the meeting. At the beginning of the meeting the physician and administrator could acknowledge their new roles and request input from the team on how the IDT has functioned.

Disease Progression

Case Study #2

Mr. Becker is a 72-year-old male with a diagnosis of prostate cancer. He received a course of radiation seven months ago and has been relatively symptom free for the past five months. His PSA was nearly normal at his last examination. When he saw the physician for a follow-up visit last week, the physician asked Mr. Becker if he had any pain. Mr. Becker said that he did. The physician did not ask where the pain was and Mr. Becker did not offer that information. The physician ordered sustained release morphine tablets 15 mg twice a day by mouth for Mr. Becker.

That night, he took his first dose and fell asleep at around midnight. At 4 AM, he awoke with abdominal pain. Again, he stated that he had "pain." His wife waited until the morning and called the doctor with the report. The physician ordered 30 mg of sustained release morphine twice a day rather than the 15 mg.

By 10 PM on that night, Mr. Becker had had 3 doses of 30 mg sustained release morphine. He still had abdominal pain. He fell asleep and then he awoke around 2 AM, yelling, very confused, and crying out with pain. His wife called 911 because she did not know what else to do.

While in the ER, the decision was made to admit Mr. Becker. A work-up revealed a bowel obstruction that turn out to be feces. He spent several days with an N/G tube in place and agents to promote peristalsis were administered. A more thorough work-up revealed:

- Constipation related to use of opiates
- Pain in bones
- Confusion related to use of sustained release products

The discharge plan was:

- Senokot S 2 tablets at bedtime
- Ibuprofen 800 mg daily for bone pain. If relief not obtained, begin prednisone
- Refer to hospice

1. Why was it important that the physician ask Mr. Becker about the location, frequency, duration, and kind of pain he was experiencing?

2. Why do opioids cause constipation?

Case Study #2 Answers

1. **Answer:** The review of this case study shows that if the physician had asked these particular questions about Mr. Becker's pain, the morphine would most likely not have been ordered. NSAIDs or steroids would have been ordered to relieve bone pain. Then, the need for laxatives would not have been as great. Note that in the initial assessment, there was no question about bowel movements. Mr. Becker should have been asked regarding prior use of opioids because sustained release pain medications should not be used on opioid-naive patients.

2. **Answer:** Opioids cause the peristalsis to slow, thereby allowing for more water to be absorbed in the colon and out of the stool, making the stool harder and thus more difficult to pass.

Disease Progression

Case Study #3

Ms. Sanders is a 55-year-old female with advanced amyotrophic lateral sclerosis. The physician referred her to hospice several weeks ago. Since then, Ms. Sanders' anxiety has increased steadily despite the administration of anxiolytics. Her biggest fear is that she will suffocate. She is an intelligent person who did research about her disease when she was first diagnosed. She has been told many times that hospice will provide the right medication to relieve her breathing problems and that the medication will probably be morphine.

1. When the patient asks about whether or not the morphine will restrict her breathing and cause her death, what is the most appropriate nursing response?

2. The family has asked hospice to help them make sure that they administer the medication as soon as possible when the patient needs it. What would be a good and cost effective way to do this?

3. The family has told the nurse that they really do not want the patient to die at home. What would be the appropriate next step?

Case Study #3 Answers

1. **Answer:** "The morphine will help ease your breathing." Morphine will relieve painful breathing by allowing the breaths to become fuller, thereby easing the strain on accessory muscles. The premise of the Principle of Double Effect is that the intention of administering a medication is never to cause or hasten death but to relieve suffering. If death occurs, that is secondary to only the intention of relief.

2. **Answer:** Talk to the registered nurse to see if the anxiolytics can be ordered as scheduled doses instead of "as needed."

3. **Answer:** Ask the family to share their feelings on this matter. Asking "why" can put people on the defensive because it may sound like a judgment. Let the family know you will take their concerns back to the team.

Pain

Case Study #4

You are a licensed practical/vocational nurse making a visit with a 40-year-old woman with metastatic breast cancer to the bone and spine. She indicates pain in two places: her right thigh and mid-back. She describes her thigh pain as a deep, dull ache that worsens when she puts weight on it while walking. She describes her mid-back pain as a shooting or burning sensation that moves down to her left thigh. Her present medication regimen is acetaminophen and oxycodone (Percocet®) 2 tablets every 3 hours around the clock. Her pain scores (on a 0–10 scale) are

Location	Pain Rating at its Best	Pain Rating at its Worst	Pain Rating Now
Right Thigh	4	8	5
Mid-Back	6	9	7

1. What additional assessment data is needed for pain management in this patient?

2. What type(s) of pain origin do you think your patient is experiencing?

3. Do you feel the patient's pain is being adequately relieved with her current regimen? What would you suggest?

4. What non-pharmacological approaches might you want to try with this patient?

Case Study #4 Answers

1. **Answer:** A better understanding about the onset and duration of pain episodes by site as well as any relieving factors would contribute to a more complete pain management regimen. Obtaining the patient's desired goals for pain management success is also important data to collect. The National Comprehensive Cancer Network's (NCCN) guidelines (2010) state that a pain score of 1–3 is mild and their goal is to keep pain levels within that range. Of course, this would take into consideration how the patient feels. This particular patient may feel a level 3 pain is acceptable, and another patient may feel as though a level 3 is too high.

2. **Answer:** The patient's right thigh pain characteristics are classic signs of bone involvement somatic pain and her mid-back pain appears to be neuropathic in origin.

3. **Answer:** The patient appears to be having minimal relief with the current regimen and seems to be experiencing constant pain as evidenced by her taking medication every 3 hours and her best pain intensity ratings are only 4 and 6. Further, the 24 hour dose of acetaminophen should not exceed 4 grams (4000 mg) for adults and the patient is consuming over 5 grams with her current regimen (each Percocet® tablet contains 325 mg acetaminophen), which can cause liver damage.

   The physician may consider adding an NSAID, changing the Percocet® to immediate release oxycodone around the clock to reduce acetaminophen toxicity and adding Neurontin starting at 100 mg at hs. Reassessment of pain relief would be needed in 24 hours and again in 48 hours. Based on pain relief with adjuvant and immediate release opioid, the physician may consider switching the oxycodone to the long-acting version OxyContin® with immediate release oxycodone for breakthrough pain. This would hopefully provide greater and consistent pain relief. The patient would need to be reassessed at 24 and 48 hours and readjust her pain medications as necessary, titrating to effect. A bowel regimen needs to be initiated at the same time.

4. **Answer:** There are many non-pharmacologic interventions that can be used concurrently with medications to relieve pain and can often be taught to patients and/or family members. Non-pharmacologic interventions should never preclude appropriate use of medications, including opioids.

   Some non-pharmacological approaches that might be appropriate for this patient may include: applying heat or cold, massage, healing touch, relaxation, guided imagery, music, aromatherapy, and TENS therapy. These are different from complementary therapies. If the patient is taking any complementary medications, they need to be sure there is no interference with the opioids.

Symptom Management

Case Study #5

Mrs. Krick is a 60-year-old female with recently diagnosed unresectable esophageal cancer, with an esophageal pleural fistula and empyema at the right pleural base. She also has a tumor near her pancreas. She presently is receiving artificial nutrition (Jevity®) through a G-tube, has a chest tube drain for the empyema, and a pigtail drain for the pleural effusion drainage.

Mrs. Krick was very involved in her work with the government and had not been able to work since the date of her diagnosis. Presenting symptoms upon seeing the doctor were unexplained intermittent belching and vomiting. She also now has continuous hiccoughing. When asked what bothers her the most, she states the hiccoughs. Present medication for this symptom is chlorproMAZINE 50mg PO q 6. Mrs. Krick states that this medication is not working and she's losing sleep and can't talk without being interrupted with hiccoughs. Her husband vouches for her comments stating that he has been sleeping in the room with her overnight. He is very supportive, as are her 2 adult children.

1. What are possible causes for her hiccoughs?

2. In performing your assessment, what would you assess for?

3. What non-pharmacologic intervention would be appropriate to treat Mrs. Krick's hiccoughs?

4. What are some of the possible pharmacologic interventions for hiccoughs?

Case Study #5 Answers

1. **Answer:** Any sort of chest surgery or trauma that directly or indirectly affects the diaphragm, can cause hiccoughs. Tumors of the neck, lung, or mediastinum by virtue of their location, can affect the diaphragm. GI disorders can involve pancreatic cancer. This patient has a tumor near the pancreas. Esophageal fistula may cause compression of sympathetic nerves producing hiccoughs. Jevity® feedings may also be a cause of the hiccoughs depending on how much she is receiving.

2. **Answer:** Assessments could include
   - Assessing for associated signs and symptoms would help with deciding whether or not it was related to the underlying disease process.
   - Assess for the relationship of the hiccoughs to sleep. Hiccoughs that stop during sleep suggest a psychogenic cause.
   - Assess for the etiology of the hiccoughs related to medical/psychological history and/or medication usage. Hiccoughs may be related to a pre-existing medical/psychological/medication condition.
   - Assessing severity and duration of current episode and previous episodes would help you to know the extent it is interrupting the patient's quality of life. Benign hiccoughs may last up to 48 hours.

3. **Answer:** Non-pharmacological treatments could include
   - Interference with normal respiratory function (holding her breath) would cause an interruption in the breathing process hopefully stopping the contractions of the diaphragm.
   - Complementary therapies such as hypnosis or acupuncture.
   - Nasopharyngeal stimulation may help stop hiccoughs through inhibiting the hiccough reflex arc.

4. **Answer:** Pharmacologic treatments based on assessment could include
   - Metoclopramide speeds up gastric motility, and also relaxes the pyloric and duodenal segments, and prevents gastroesophageal reflux.
   - Baclofen decreases neurotransmitter function and decreases the frequency and severity of muscle spasms.
   - ChlorproMAZINE is a centrally acting tranquilizer and dopamine antagonist. Frequently reassess for effectiveness and be sure that side effects do not outweigh benefits.

Communication

Case Study #6

Mrs. Kim is an 87-year-old widow dying of metastatic ovarian cancer. She is living at home and receiving hospice care. Her two middle-aged daughters take turns providing physical care. Her son also is involved in her care. The team is finding it difficult to work with him because he insists on making all the decisions for his mother even though she is alert and oriented. Mrs. Kim speaks limited English. Her daughters and son are fluent in English and Korean.

1. Mrs. Kim's son insists that no one on the healthcare team mention the word "cancer" or "death" to his mother. What does this request most likely reflect?

2. During one of your visits, Mrs. Kim tells you that she met her husband last night at the airport and he invited her home. What would be the most appropriate response to Mrs. Kim?

3. You are helping one of the daughters change Mrs. Kim's position and you notice the daughter is crying. She tells you that taking care of her mother is very difficult. What would be the most appropriate response to the daughter?

Case Study #6 Answers

1. **Answer:** Many cultures believe that open discussion about death and illness is rude and harmful. Some cultures also believe that it can destroy the patient's hope and hasten death.

2. **Answer:** Ask Mrs. Kim to tell you more about the experience. Mrs. Kim's comments may reflect symbolic language used by some dying patients. Asking her to tell you more about the experience can give you clues about Mrs. Kim's readiness for death and meaning that the event has for her. Reminding Mrs. Kim that her husband died may only upset her. The focus should not be on confirming or discounting her story. Instead, explore the meaning that the story has for her. Mrs. Kim's comments do not necessarily indicate delirium; thus, changing her medication may cause unnecessary problems. Mrs. Kim's comments do not necessarily reflect organ failure. Drawing blood to check lab values is an inappropriate way to respond to her experience and discounts the importance of its meaning to her.

3. **Answer:** After completing Mrs. Kim's physical care, encourage her to tell you more about her feelings. Encourage families to express their feelings. Allowing the daughter to talk also will clarify what specifically she finds difficult (e.g., emotions, physical care, role strain) and assist the team in identifying ways to assist the daughter. The daughter has provided you an opening for discussion of her feelings. Explore her emotions and needs more fully before suggesting she talk with the social worker. Then ask her if she would like to talk with a social worker to discuss what she is feeling right now and what she has shared with you.

Culture

Case Study #7

Mrs. Chin is a 75-year-old Chinese American who is hospitalized with colon cancer. This is her second day in the hospital. Mrs. Chin has three daughters and two sons who live in the same state. For the past eight years Mrs. Chin has been living with one of her daughters. Mrs. Chin prepared the meals and did light housekeeping for her daughter. She enjoys hot Ginseng tea in the morning and in the evening. Mrs. Chin drank an herbal preparation for a "tonic" in the morning. Her daughter asks you if she can continue to have Ginseng tea and her tonic. Mrs. Chin informs you that she is in the hospital because she had problems with her "bowels." She asks you if the doctors have found out what is wrong with her. You note a comment in the medical record that the family is aware of the diagnosis, but have asked that Mrs. Chin not be told she has cancer. Mrs. Chin looks uncomfortable, she is frowning and grimaces with movement. You ask Mrs. Chin if she would like some medication for pain, but she denies having any pain.

1. Mrs. Chin's family has requested that she not be informed of her diagnosis. You plan to talk to the physician about this request. What is a possible explanation?

2. Mrs. Chin's daughter asks if it is okay to bring her mother's tonic in to the hospital. What is the most appropriate response to this request?

3. Mrs. Chin has signs of pain, yet when you ask her if she is experiencing pain she denies it. You explain to Mrs. Chin that you can give her some medication to make her more comfortable. What might be Mrs. Chin's reasons for not complaining of pain?

Case Study #7 Answers

1. **Answer:** Many Asian cultural groups believe informing a person of a cancer diagnosis takes away hope. It is common in many Asian cultural groups to believe that informing a person of a serious illness takes away hope. Although it is important to recognize that this may not apply to all Asian Americans.

2. **Answer:** Ask the daughter to bring in some tonic so it can be determined if the tonic would cause any interactions with medications. The primary concern about tonics or herbal medications is that that may result in drug interactions. The tonic may interact with some of the medications, therefore it should be determined if it may cause any drug interactions.

3. **Answer:** She may believe that pain should be endured and she should not complain. The response to pain varies in cultural groups. She may also be fearful of addiction or believe that medication should only be given for severe pain, but the most logical explanation may be due to a cultural response. The word pain itself may be a barrier, try other words like discomfort and hurt, or words that describe the pain (e.g., throbbing, aching, and stabbing).

Spirituality

Case Study #8

Mrs. Yates has been a very optimistic resident with a good sense of humor. Everyone on the team has commented on how well she is handling her terminal illness and the fact that she can no longer live alone. During Mrs. Yates' morning bath at the nursing home, she begins crying and tells you how lonely she is. She says no one ever comes to visit her, and she is especially hurt that the minister of the church she attended when living at home does not visit her. She says she wishes she could talk with her sister who lives in another state and cannot travel because of her own illness. She begins talking about her son who was killed in a motor vehicle accident when he was 17 and tells you that she is ready to see him again. She asks you why she is still alive as she thinks her life no longer has any purpose.

1. What would be your best immediate response to Mrs. Yates?

2. What else should you do in response to this interaction with Mrs. Yates?

3. How would you respond to Mrs. Yates' question about why she is alive when her life has no purpose?

Case Study #8 Answers

1. **Answer:** The best thing you can do is to be a good listener and allow Mrs. Yates to discuss the things which are causing her such emotional pain. Although she has been optimistic and happy up to this point, you should realize that dying patients often have spiritual and emotional concerns as they get closer to death. You might ask a few questions to show your interest and encourage her to explore her feelings. You would not rush her or tell her you are too busy. While you might be tempted to cheer Mrs. Yates by ignoring the things that are upsetting her and telling her that the team likes her and her usually cheerful personality, this would not be helpful to her because she is dealing with some deep feelings about her life, her death, and those she has loved. By remaining present with her and allowing her to be sad and tell you about her feelings, you are helping her with her spiritual concerns.

2. **Answer:** You should ask Mrs. Yates how you and your team can best help her. Would she like for someone to contact her minister? Would she like a visit from the chaplain? Could someone help her to contact her sister by phone or letter? After you have listened well and talked with her about her feelings and needs, you should report to the team. The team should use this information to develop or change the plan of care for this patient so that it deals with her spiritual needs and concerns. The team can decide on the best member to help her with her concerns, or it may be that several members have a role. For instance, you might help her write a letter to her sister or make a phone call while the chaplain makes a visit to her to meet her needs for pastoral care or help her connect with the minister from her church. Perhaps a volunteer can be assigned to Mrs. Yates so that she is not so alone and has someone to talk with about her life.

3. **Answer:** This is a question about the meaning of life that has no answer. You might ask Mrs. Yates why she thinks she is still alive or have her think about what she can do to give some meaning to the rest of her life. You might encourage her to share more about her past or her son as reviewing her life might help her to find meaning in her existence. You should help Mrs. Yates explore her own feelings rather than telling her what you believe about the meaning of life or trying to get her to see things as you do.

Pediatric

Case Study #9a

Crystal is a 5-year-old little girl with spinal muscular atrophy (SMA), whose illness has been progressing rapidly in the last 2 months. SMA is the second most common autosomal recessive disease in Caucasians; pathology includes degeneration of the spinal anterior horn cells, atrophy and wasting of skeletal muscles. There are three types: SMA I is also known as Werdnig-Hoffman disease, which is rapidly progressive with death usually occurring by 3 years of age; SMA II is the intermediate form progressing more slowly with many children living to school age; SMA III is also known as Kugelberg-Welander disease, which is slowly progressive and these children may actually reach adulthood. The usual presentations include: floppy baby, arthrogrypsos, muscle weakness in infancy, weakness and wasting. Crystal has been diagnosed with Stage 1 to Stage 2, meaning that her disease is not as aggressive as most Stage 1s but progressing more rapidly than most Stage 2s.

Currently Crystal is not able to swallow and is fed by bolus G-tube feedings during the day with continuous feedings at night, she is on BiPAP at night with frequent nebulizer treatments during the day and is oxygen dependent on 2–10 liters/hour. She has had three different hospitalizations in the last 8 weeks, each admission for pneumonia and increasing respiratory difficulties requiring intubation and intensive care. Each hospitalization has resulted in increased respiratory needs, with greater difficulty weaning her off of the ventilator. Crystal is cognitively intact however her physical status has declined to the point where she is now unable to move anything but her right arm with only gross motor skills in her right hand. Since diagnosis, Crystal has spent much of her 5 years in the hospital with repeated pneumonias, having grown up in an adult world Crystal is "older than her years."

1. Crystal states that she hurts "too much." Based on Crystal's developmental level what is the best way to assess her pain?

2. The pediatrician has recommended changing Crystal's pain medication to an opioid. Her mother is concerned about giving Crystal medication that is "too strong" for her. How would you respond to her mother's concerns?

Case Study #9a Answers

1. **Answer:** At the age of 5 Crystal would be considered preschool, but given that she is considered "older than her years," some of the aspects of a school-age child might also apply to her.
   - Preschool child: allow Crystal to try out the equipment, give her choices, allow her to help, make sure her Mom is close by, give positive reinforcement, be aware that she may have some stranger anxiety, find out what words she uses to describe her pain and include her in the assessment and any decisions that are made.
   - School-age child: use simple explanations regarding her illness, ask if she knows what causes her pain; answer any of her questions honestly and briefly. Ask what she thinks should be done about her pain. Use her words to describe her pain. Picture books may help. Offer choices.

2. **Answer:** Children can take many of the same pain medications that an adult can take. Working with the registered nurse and pharmacist, the pediatrician will order pain medications for Crystal that are appropriate for children and will assure that it is the correct dosage that is based on Crystal's weight.

Pediatric

Case Study #9b

Crystal's mother (from Case Study #9a) is a single parent, 25-years-old, with an extended family. Crystal has three siblings ages 2, 7, and 10. Mom has a high school education, which is the highest level of education of any family member. Mom and family members' experience with the healthcare community had been restricted to childbirth and well baby visits until Crystal's illness was diagnosed at 9 months of age.

Crystal is now being discharged to home with home health. Up until this admission, each time Crystal's condition changed in any way, her Mom rushed her to the emergency room. Mom has been unable to discuss Crystal's deteriorating condition or her prognosis. Whenever a member of the healthcare team initiates discussion about a plan of care for Crystal she breaks down in tears and leaves the room. Crystal, on the other hand, keeps indicating that she only wants to be at home and tries to prevent any interventions by swatting at the team member. She has clearly communicated with the healthcare team in Mom's presence that she knows that she will die and go to heaven if they don't put the tube in her throat and that she is tired. Crystal states "My body isn't good here anymore and I want to go to heaven and be with grandma. I'm tired and I hurt too much."

The healthcare team has scheduled a patient care conference with Mom to discuss discharge planning. Attending the conference is the primary physician, a pediatric pulmonologist who has taken care of Crystal since diagnosis as well as the nurse case manager, the hospital social worker, the hospital chaplain, the chief resident, the home care service case manager and the staff nurse taking care of Crystal. Mom is alone with the 2-year-old sibling.

1. There has been no attempt to discuss goals of care with Crystal or her mother since last admission when Mom left the room in tears when the subject of a pre-hospital DNR was brought up. All patient care conferences up to this point have consisted of the primary physician and the nurse case manager. What, if anything, do you see as a problem with the make-up of those attending this patient care conference for discharge planning?

2. Clearly Crystal is ready for a DNR and Mom is not. What can be done to help bridge the gap between mother and daughter?

3. Mom's coping until this admission has been to bring Crystal back to the emergency room. What can the nurse do during discharge teaching to empower Mom to keep Crystal at home as long as possible?

Case Study #9b Answers

1. **Answer:** Mom may feel threatened and overwhelmed alone in the room with so many. Although child life should be part of the team, this team is way too big and overwhelming for this young mother who has no one with her but her 2-year-old son. For the first meeting 2 to 3 team members should meet with the Mom to initiate the discussion, outline the assessment and goals of the healthcare team, and learn Mom's CURRENT level of understanding and goals for her daughter and family. At the end of the initial meeting another meeting can be scheduled with the other members of the healthcare team that are necessary OR Mom can be asked if she would like to meet with any of the other team members.

2. **Answer:** A team member, usually the nurse, close to both Mom and Crystal can help facilitate a discussion with both of them present to address their goals for care. Whenever possible, incorporating the child along with the family in the decision-making is best. Our job is to work WITH the child and family in defining their goals and assisting them in how to best meet them. Mom has never given any indication that she is not capable and although her coping may not be what we want it does not equate with being wrong.

3. **Answers** can include
   - Introduce hospice staff before discharge.
   - Include specific instructions for pain and symptom management.
   - Provide a 24/7 contact number for telephone support and assistance.
   - Explain the different scenarios that may occur in the home with Crystal and work through the appropriate responses for each.
   - Include Crystal in the teaching and have both Mom and Crystal decide the desired plan and outcomes.

   All answers support empowering primary caregiver and child in the decision-making process. This is a wonderful opportunity to focus on "doing for" rather than "doing to" Crystal.

Family Caregivers

Case Study #10

Mrs. Hays is a 60-year-old woman with widely metastatic breast cancer. She is living at home with her husband John, age 64, and recently just started receiving hospice. Her husband and a friend care for her around the clock. As her disease worsens, her husband begins calling hospice several times a day for help and reassurance.

1. Even though Mr. Hays has demonstrated understanding and competence in providing her care, he becomes afraid that he will do something wrong and become the cause of her death. What does Mr. Hays' behavior most likely reflect?

2. During one of your visits to the home, Mr. Hays shares that he feels lonely and isolated from the world. What is the best response to Mr. Hays?

3. A friend of Mr. Hays' shares with you his concern over a recent conversation they had. Mr. Hays is struggling with his faith and is angry at God for his wife's illness. What is the best explanation for this to give his friend?

Case Study #10 Answers

1. **Answer:** It reflects the need for emotional validation and encouragement for the good job he is doing in caring for his wife. Mr. Hays is calling because he's feeling uncertain and inadequate, even though he is doing a very good job in caring for his wife. Validating his feelings and then moving him on by words of encouragement will help put his mind at ease. He has already demonstrated an ability to care for his wife. His feelings are common among family caregivers; therefore do not warrant psychological help.

2. **Answer:** "Mr. Hays, in many ways you are isolated from life as you knew it; it is understandable that you would feel lonely." Acknowledge his feelings and in doing so, you are validating him as a person. Responses should not minimize his feelings, thereby invalidating his personhood and adding to his sense of loneliness. Remember, feelings are neither right nor wrong. They just are.

3. **Answer:** "It is not uncommon for someone's faith to be shaken during a time like this. The best thing to do is just be there to listen, not to judge." Listening provides the greatest intervention during these times. Most people just need the freedom to be angry at God and vent their feelings without being judged. You don't want to say anything that would be a judgment on his faith. Enlightening the friend about what he is already doing and then validating him, is the best response.

Bereavement

Case Study #11

Mrs. Clark, a 55-year-old woman with stage IV ovarian cancer, had recently finished the last treatments available for her disease and the CA-125 was once again on the rise. She had coped well with great support from her family over the past 3 years. Within a week of learning there was nothing more that could be done; she received news that her 7-year-old granddaughter was killed in a car accident while accompanying her father on his errands. This was her only grandchild with whom she shared a special bond. Mrs. Clark's son-in-law was taken to the hospital in serious condition, but will be fine. The Clarks decide to go on hospice because Mrs. Clark needs help with symptom management. During one of the hospice visits, Mr. Clark shares that his wife is becoming more depressed and tearful and that is not normal for her. He understands she is sad, but feels helpless in knowing what to do for her.

1. What does Mrs. Clark's behavior reflects?

2. During one of your visits, the Clarks' daughter shares that she doesn't know if she can handle all that is going on—her mother's going to die, she just lost her only child, and her husband is in the hospital. What is this daughter at risk for?

3. Mrs. Clark is doing poorly and is now bedridden. Mr. Clark shares that she has been having very unusual experiences where she waves to the air like she's waving at someone, and then she says she sees John. John is her brother who died when he was young from whooping cough. It's almost like she is lucid but if you try to talk to her, she doesn't really make sense. What is your best explanation/ response to Mr. Clark?

Case Study #11 Answers

1. **Answer:** Bereavement. Mrs. Clark has just experienced a personal loss in learning there is nothing else that can be done for her cancer. She will succumb to the disease and die. She also loses her only granddaughter with whom she was very close. She is experiencing a complex series of reactions following death—death in different forms.

2. **Answer:** Complicated grief. This daughter is at risk for complicated grief due to the sudden and traumatic death of her daughter and the impending death of her mother, not to mention that her closest support is in the hospital recovering from the accident.

3. **Answer:** This is a common experience for patients who are close to death and they are not hallucinations. What she is experiencing will not hurt her and these experiences usually help provide a peaceful death. Unless there is a physiological reason for hallucinations or delirium, there is no reason to try to "treat" the unusual experience.

Time of Dying

Case Study #12

Mr. Davis, a hospice patient in a long-term care facility, became unresponsive last night. His wife has been visiting daily, and now expresses concern that Mr. Davis is suffering, because he has been restless today from time to time. Mrs. Davis says she is most upset that her husband can no longer communicate with her, stating "I knew he was dying, but I thought we would have more time to talk together."

1. What are the most likely causes of Mr. Davis's restlessness?

2. What are some nursing actions that may make Mr. Davis comfortable?

3. List some examples of role-modeling that nurses can do to impact on Mr. Davis's care.

4. Identify several ways to provide support to Mr. Davis's wife at this time.

Case Study #12 Answers

1. **Answer:** The most likely causes of Mr. Davis's restlessness could be terminal delirium, full bladder, constipation and/or fecal impaction, wet or soiled linens from incontinence, or sweating. Other causes could be physical pain, or spiritual distress.

2. **Answer:** Nursing actions are to
   - Determine if Mr. Davis has a full bladder, fecal impaction, or constipation.
   - Ensure clean, dry bed linens that are not wrinkled under him.
   - Observe Mr. Davis's response to environmental changes such as room lighting, presence of visitors, response to the care provided.
   - Turn Mr. Davis at frequent intervals and support his positions, check for pressure areas or other skin breakdown.
   - Observe and report if Mr. Davis has furrowing of the brow, which may indicate true pain.
   - Observe and report Mr. Davis's response to pain or other medications that are given.

3. **Answer:** Examples of role-modeling for family and other caretakers are
   - Talking to Mr. Davis any time you are in the room, telling him who you are and what you are going to do.
   - Orient Mr. Davis to place and time.
   - Avoid conversations with others in the room that do NOT include Mr. Davis—assume that he can hear, and include him in any conversations.
   - Attempt alternate communication with Mr. Davis from time to time, asking him to respond by blinking or squeezing a hand to a yes or no question, as responsiveness may alter from time to time.

4. **Answer:** Providing support to Mr. Davis's wife includes
   - Listening and responding to her concerns.
   - Being frequently present and attentive to the care of Mr. Davis.
   - Report to Mrs. Davis, her husband's status and what has been done for him when she is not at his bedside.
   - Helping Mrs. Davis identify available support such as her family, friends, clergy, etc.
   - Referring Mrs. Davis to a social worker, clergy, or other counselor who can be helpful to the grieving process.
   - Providing information about the normal grieving process.

Professional Development

Case Study #13

Patrick, a licensed practical nurse, has been working at a long-term care agency for the past three years on a 40-bed-unit on the evening shift. The residents on this unit have chronic debilitating illnesses. He is responsible for the medication administration for the 40-bed-unit and supervision of the nursing assistants. He also evaluates the residents each shift and reports problems to the registered nurse supervisor.

Mrs. O'Keefe has been a resident on the unit for three years. Her cardiac condition is failing rapidly. Based on Mrs. O'Keefe's advance directives, which her family supports, Mrs. O'Keefe will remain on the unit until she dies. She is being seen by hospice, who are directing her supportive care.

1. Patrick has been asked by the son of Mrs. O'Keefe's roommate "There is something obviously wrong with her, why aren't you doing anything? Are you going to just let her die?" Patrick explains that he understands his concern for Mrs. O'Keefe, but cannot give him information about Mrs. O'Keefe's condition, but assured him the staff is following the care requested by the patient and her family. Patrick also asks him if he and his mother ever discussed her end-of-life wishes. Which behaviors of professionalism is Patrick following?

2. Mrs. O'Keefe has developed dyspnea due to an accumulation of fluid in her lungs. She is not taking in anything by mouth. Her physician has ordered for her to have IV furosemide and morphine to decrease the dyspnea. The registered nurse supervisor starts the IV on Mrs. O'Keefe and instructs Patrick to give the IV medications as she is very busy that evening and will not have time. Patrick knows that according to his state's nurse practice act he is not permitted to give IV push medications. How should Patrick respond to the supervisor's request?

3. Mrs. O'Keefe's family tells Patrick that on his next day off they would like to take him out to dinner to thank him for the good care that he has been giving Mrs. O'Keefe. By politely declining their offer, Patrick is exhibiting what aspect of professional growth and development.

Case Study #13 Answers

1. **Answer:** These are some of the possible answers, you may have others.
   - Altruism—he has put Mrs. O'Keefe and her family first and advocated for her by assuring that her wishes are being followed.
   - Integrity—he answered the son truthfully.
   - Caring/compassion/communication—he listened to the son and guided the conversation to determine if the son and his mother have talked about her end-of-life wishes.
   - Respect—he respected Mrs. O'Keefe's privacy by not giving away personal information.
   - Responsibility/accountability—by controlling his emotions when talking to the son who was confrontational.
   - Excellence/scholarship—he is committed to providing the best care he can.
   - Leadership—he has followed the standards of care and standards of professional behavior as designated by the specialty.

2. **Answer:** Following his state's nurse practice act guidelines, Patrick needs to remind his supervisor that as a licensed practical/vocational nurse, he is not permitted to give IV push medications and therefore cannot do as she asks. He can ask her if there is another registered nurse who is working the evening shift that can give the medication.

3. **Answer:** Maintaining professional boundaries.

General References

Abrahm JL. Update in palliative medicine and end-of-life care. *Annu Rev Med.* 2003;54:53–72.

Amenta MO, Bohnet NL, eds. *Nursing Care of the Terminally Ill.* Boston, MA: Little, Brown and Company; 1986.

American Association of Colleges of Nursing and the City of Hope National Medical Center. *End-of-Life Nursing Education Consortium (ELNEC) Project.* 2010. Funded through the Robert Wood Johnson Foundation.

American Geriatrics Society, Adler R, Kame H. *Doorway Thoughts: Cross-Cultural Health Care for Older Adults.* Boston, MA: Jones & Bartlett Publishers; 2004.

American Psychiatric Association. *Diagnostic and Statistical Manual of Mental Disorders.* 4th ed. Washington, DC: American Psychiatric Association; 2000.

Anderson KO, Green CR, Payne R. Racial and ethnic disparities in pain: causes and consequences of unequal care. *J Pain.* 2009;10(12):1187–1204.

Andrews MM, Boyle JS, eds. *Transcultural Concepts in Nursing Care.* 5th ed. Philadelphia, PA: Lippincott; 2008.

Benjamin LJ, Dampler CD, Jacox A, et al. *Guidelines for the Management of Acute and Chronic Pain in Sickle-Cell Disease.* Skokie, IL: American Pain Society; 1999.

Bergstrom N, et al., *Pressure Ulcer Treatment: Clinical Practice Guideline. Quick Reference Guide for Clinicians, No. 15.* Rockville, MD: U.S. Department of Health and Human Services, Public Health Service, Agency for Health Care Policy and Research; 1994.

Berry PH, ed. *Core Curriculum for the Generalist Hospice and Palliative Nurse.* 3rd ed. Dubuque, IA: Kendall Hunt; 2010.

Borneman T. Caring for cancer patients at home: the effect on family caregivers. *Home Health Care Manag Pract.* 1998;10(4):25–33.

Bowlby J. *Attachment and Loss.* New York, NY: Basic Books; 1980.

Brashers VL. Alterations in pulmonary function. In: McCance KL, Huether SE, eds. *Pathophysiology: The Biologic Basis for Disease in Adults and Children.* 4th ed. St. Louis, MO: Mosby; 2002:1105–1144.

Brenner R. Hospice care and palliative care: a perspective from experience. *Hosp J.* 1999;14(3/4):155–166.

Brown-Saltzman K. Transforming the grief experience. In: Carroll-Johnson RM, Gorman L, Bush N, eds. *Psychosocial Nursing Care along the Cancer Continuum.* Pittsburgh, PA: Oncology Nursing Press, Inc.; 2006:293–314.

Byock I. *Dying well: The Prospects for Growth at the End of Life.* New York, NY: Riverhead Books; 1997.

Byock IR. Hospice and palliative care: a parting of the ways or a path to the future. *J Palliat Med.* 1998;1: 165–176.

Callanan M, Kelley P. *Final Gifts: Understanding the Special Awareness, Needs, & Communications of the Dying.* New York, NY: Bantam Books; 1997.

Campbell T, Hately J. The management of nausea and vomiting in advanced cancer. *Int J Palliat Nurs.* 2000;6(1):18–20, 22–25.

Center for Advancement of Palliative Care. *Designing a Palliative Care Team.* Available at: www.capc.org/building-a-hospital-based-palliative-care-program/index_html. Accessed July 6, 2009.

Centers for Disease Control and Prevention, National Center for Health Statistics. *National Vital Statistics Report.* 2009. Available at: www.cdc.gov/nchs/data/nvsr/nvsr57/nvsr57_14.pdf. Accessed February 2, 2010.

Children's Hospice International. *Children's Hospice International: 2001 Informational Overview.* Alexandria, VA: 2001, Children's Hospice International; 2001.

Chochinov HM, Breitbart W. *Handbook of Psychiatry in Palliative Care.* 2nd ed. New York, NY: Oxford University Press; 2009.

Clark E. *Palliative Pain and Symptom Management for Children and Adolescents.* Children's Hospice International and Division of Maternal and Child Health—U.S. Department of Health and Human Services: Alexandria, VA; 1985.

Cleelan C, et al. Pain and its treatment in outpatients with metastatic cancer. *N Engl J Med.* 1994;330: 592–596.

Collins CA. Ascites. *Clin J Oncol Nurs.* 2001;5(1):43–44.

Conner SR. New initiatives transforming hospice care. *Hosp J.* 1999;14(3/4):193–203.

Corr CA, Nabe CM, Corr DM. *Death and Dying: Live and Living.* 6th ed. Belmont, CA: Thomson/Wadsworth; 2008.

Dahlin C, Lentz J, Sutermaster DJ. *Competencies for the Hospice and Palliative Licensed Practical/Vocational Nurse.* 2nd ed. Dubuque, IA: Kendall Hunt Professional; 2009.

Dahlin C, Lentz J, Sutermaster DJ. *Statement of the Scope and Standards of Hospice and Palliative Licensed Practical/Vocational Nursing Practice.* Dubuque, IA: Kendall Hunt Publishing Company; 2004.

Deming WE. *Out of the Crisis.* Cambridge, MA: Massachusetts Institute of Technology Center for Advanced Engineering Study; 1986.

Doyle D, Hanks G, Macdonald N, eds. *Oxford Textbook of Palliative Medicine.* Oxford, UK: Oxford Medical Publication; 2009.

Drought TS, Koening BA. "Choice" in end of life decision-making: research fact or fiction? *Gerontologist.* 2002;42(Special Issue III):114–128.

Duhamel F, Dupuis F. Guaranteed returns: investing in conversations with families of patients with cancer. *Clin J Oncol Nurs.* 2004;8(1):68–71.

Duke S. An exploration of anticipatory grief: the lived experience of people during their spouses' terminal illness and in bereavement. *J Adv Nurs.* 1998;28(4):829–839.

Eastern Cooperative Oncology Group. *ECOG Performance Status.* 2006. Available at: www.ecog.org/general/perf_stat.html. Accessed February 3, 2010.

El-Jawahri AR, Prigerson HG. Bereavement care. In: Berger A, Portenoy R, Weissman D, eds. *Principles & Practice of Palliative Care & Supportive Oncology.* 3rd ed. Philadelphia, PA: Lippincott Williams & Wilkins; 2007:645–653.

Erikson E. *Childhood and Society.* New York, NY: W.W. Norton & Co.; 1963.

Ersek M. Artificial nutrition and hydration: clinical issues. *J Hosp Palliat Care*. 2003;5(4):221–230.

Fairchild A. Undertreatment of cancer pain. *Curr Opin Support Palliat Care*. 2010;4(1):11–15.

Farber SJ, Egnew TR, Herman-Bertsch JL, Taylor TR, Guldin GE. Issues in end-of-life care: patient, caregiver, and clinician perceptions. *J Palliat Med*. 2003;6(1):19–31.

Farran CJ, Herth KA, Popovich JM. *Hope and Hopelessness: Critical Clinical Concepts*. Thousand Oaks, CA: Sage; 1995.

Fehring RJ, Miller JF, Shaw C. Spiritual well-being, religiosity, hope, depression, and other mood states in elderly people coping with cancer. *Oncol Nurs Forum*. 1997;24:663–671.

Ferrell BR, Coyle N, eds. *Textbook of Palliative Nursing*. 3rd ed. New York, NY: Oxford University Press; 2010.

Ferszt B, Houck P. The family. In: Amenta MO, Bohnet NL, eds. *Nursing Care of the Terminally Ill*. Boston, MA: Little, Brown and Company; 1986:173–190.

Field MJ, Cassel CK. *Approaching Death: Improving Care at the End of Life*. Washington, DC: Institute of Medicine Task Force; 1997.

Foley G. *Lessons from the Bereaved: Care for the Dying*. Paper presented at the Sixth National Conference on Cancer Nursing, Seattle, WA; 1991.

Fong CM. Ethnicity and nursing practice. *Top Clin Nurs*. 1985;7(3):1–10.

Forte AL, Hill M, Pazder R, Feudtner C. Bereavement care interventions: a systematic review. *BMC Palliat Care*. 2004;3(1):3.

Friebert S. *NHPCO Facts and Figures: Pediatric Palliative and Hospice Care in America*. Washington, DC: National Hospice and Palliative Care Organization; 2009.

Galanti G. *Caring for Patients from Different Cultures*. 4th ed. Philadelphia, PA: University of Pennsylvania Press; 2008.

Geriatric Interdisciplinary Team Training Curriculum. Topic 1: Teams and Teamwork. Available at: www.americangeriatrics.org/education/gitt/_topic.pdf. Accessed June 6, 2009.

Geriatric Interdisciplinary Team Training Curriculum. Topic 3: Team Communication and Conflict Resolution. Available at: www.americangeriatrics.org/education/gitt/_topic.pdf. Accessed July 7, 2009.

Gibbon MB. Psychosocial aspects of serious illness in childhood and adolescence: responding to the storm. In: Armstrong-Daily A, Zarbock S, eds. *Hospice Care for Children*. 3rd ed. New York, NY: Oxford University Press; 2009:54–75.

Giger JM, Davidhizar RE, eds. *Transcultural Nursing: Assessment & Intervention*. 4th ed. St. Louis, MO: Mobsy, Inc.; 2004:3–19.

Goldman A. ABC of palliative care: special problems of children. *BMJ*. 1998;316:49–52.

Gorman L. The psychosocial impact of cancer on the individual, family, and society. In: Carroll-Johnson RM, Gorman L, Bush N, eds. *Psychosocial Nursing Care along the Cancer Continuum*. Pittsburgh, PA: Oncology Nursing Press, Inc.; 2006:3–23.

Grunfeld E, Coyle D, Whelan T, et al. Family caregiver burden: results of a longitudinal study of breast cancer patients and their principal caregivers. *Cmaj*. 2004;170(12):1795–1801.

Hallenbeck JL. *Palliative Care Perspectives*. New York, NY: Oxford University Press; 2003.

Harding R, Higginson IJ. What is the best way to help caregivers in cancer and palliative care? A systematic literature review of interventions and their effectiveness. *Palliat Med.* 2003;17(1):63–74.

Herth K. Fostering hope in terminally-ill people. *J Adv Nurs.* 1990;15:1250–1259.

Herth K. Hope in the family caregiver of terminally-ill people. *J Adv Nurs.* 1993;18:538–548.

Herth KA, Cutcliffe JR. The concept of hope in nursing 3: hope and palliative care nursing. *Br J Nurs.* 2002;11(14):977–983.

Heubi JE, Barbacci MB, Zimmerman HJ. Therapeutic misadventures with acetaminophen: hepatoxicity after multiple doses in children. *J Pediatr.* 1998;132(1):22–27.

Hileman JW, Lackey NR. Self-identified needs of patients with cancer at home and their home caregivers: a descriptive study. *Oncol Nurs Forum.* 1990;17(6):907–913.

Huff SM, Hutton N. Pain and symptom management. In: Armstrong-Daily A, Zarbock S, eds. *Hospice Care for Children.* 3rd ed. New York, NY: Oxford University Press; 2009:24–53.

Institute of Medicine (U.S.). Committee on Communication for Behavior Change in the 21st Century: Improving the Health of Diverse Populations. *Speaking of Health: Assessing Health Communication Strategies for Diverse Populations.* Washington, DC: National Academies Press; 2002.

Isaksen AS, Thuen F, Hanestad B. Patients with cancer and their close relatives: experiences with treatment, care, and support. *Cancer Nurs.* 2003;26(1):68–74.

Jacox A, Carr DB, Payne R, et al. *Management of Cancer Pain. Clinical Practice Guideline No. 9.* AHCPR Publication No. 94-0592. Rockville, MD: Agency for Health Care Policy and Research, U.S. Department of Health and Human Services, Public Health Service; March 1994.

Jenko M, Moffitt SR. Transcultural nursing principles: an application to hospice care. *J Hosp Palliat Nurs.* 2006;8(3):172–180.

Jones RE, Huether SE. Alterations in hormonal regulation. In: McCance KL, Huether SE, eds. *Pathophysiology: The Biologic Basis for Disease in Adults and Children.* St. Louis, MO: Mosby; 2002:624–669.

Kalina K. *Midwife for Souls: Spiritual Care for the Dying.* Boston, MA: St. Paul Books and Media; 2007.

Karnofsky Performance Scale Index. Available at: www.hospicepatients.org/karnofsky.html. Accessed February 3, 2010.

Kashrut: Jewish Dietary Laws. Available at: www.jewfaq.org/kashrut.htm. Accessed February 8, 2010.

Kastenbaum RJ. *Death, Society and Human Experience.* 10th ed. Upper Saddle River, NJ: Pearson Education, Inc.; 2008.

Keene N. *Childhood Leukemia: A Guide for Families, Friends, and Caregivers.* 3rd ed. Sebastol, CA: O'Reilly & Associates, Inc; 2002:1–13.

Kemp C. *Terminal Illness: A Guide to Nursing Care.* 2nd ed. Philadelphia, PA: Lippincott; 1999.

Kubic A, Burda AM, Bockewitz E, Wahl M. Hepatotoxicity in an infant following supratherapeutic dosing of acetaminophen for twenty-four hours. *Semin Diagn Pathol.* 2009;26(1):7–9.

Kübler-Ross E. *On Death and Dying.* New York, NY: Macmillan; 1969.

Letizia M, Norton E. Successful management of malignant bowel obstruction. *J Hosp Palliat Nurs.* 2002; 5(3):152–158.

Lo K, Causey B, Crandall F. *Care at the Time of Death.* Paper presented at the Hospice Training Program, Largo, FL; 1996.

Loney M. Death, dying, and grief in the face of cancer. In: Burke C, ed. *Psychosocial Dimensions of Oncology Nursing Care*. Pittsburgh, PA: Oncology Nursing Press, Inc.; 1998:152–179.

Lynn J, Schuster JL, Kabcenel A. *Improving Care for the End of Life*. New York, NY: Oxford University Press; 2000.

Mansen TJ, McCance KL. Alterations in leukocyte, lymphoid and hemostatic function. In: McCance KL, Huether SE, eds. *Pathophysiology: The Biologic Basis for Disease in Adults and Children*. 4th ed. St. Louis, MO: Mosby; 2002:865–899.

Martsolf DS, Mickely JR. The concept of spirituality in nursing theories: differing world views and extent of focus. *J Adv Nurs*. 1998;27:294–303.

Matzo M, Sherman DW, eds. *Palliative Care Nursing: Quality Care to the End of Life*. 3rd ed. New York, NY: Springer Publishing; 2010.

McCaffery M, Pasero C. *Pain: Clinical Manual*. St. Louis, MO: Mosby; 1999.

Miller K, Miller M. Managing common gastrointestinal symptoms at the end of life. *J Hosp Palliat Nurs*. 2002;4(1):34–42.

National Board of Medical Examiners. The Behaviors of Professionalism. Available at: http://ci.nbme.org/professionalism/behaviors.asp. Accessed September 8, 2009.

National Consensus Project for Quality Palliative Care. *Clinical Practice Guidelines for Quality Palliative Care*. 2nd ed. 2009. Available at: www.nationalconsensusproject.org. Accessed February 2, 2010.

National Hospice Organization. *A Pathway for Patients and Families Facing Terminal Illness*. Arlington, VA: National Hospice Organization; 1997:5–6.

Nelson EC, Batalden PB, Ryer JC, eds. *Joint Commission Clinical Improvement Action Guide*. Oakbrook Terrace, IL: The Joint Accreditation of Healthcare Organizations; 1998.

NHPCO. *Standards of Practice for Pediatric Palliative Care and Hospice, Children's Project on Palliative/Hospice Services (ChiPPS)*. Washington DC: NHPCO; 2009:36.

North American Nursing Diagnosis Association. *Nursing Diagnoses: Definitions and Classification*. Philadelphia, PA: North American Nursing Diagnosis Association; 2007–2008.

O'Connor P. Hospice vs. palliative care. *Hosp J*. 1999;14(3/4):123–137.

Petrillo M, Sanger S. *Emotional Care of Hospitalized Children: An Environmental Approach*. 2nd ed. Philadelphia, PA: J. B. Lippincott; 1980.

Portenoy PR. *Defining Palliative Care*. Beth Israel Medical Center: Newsletter, Department of Pain and Palliative Care; 1998.

Purnell LD, Paulanka BJ. Transcultural diversity and health care. In: Purnell LD, Paulanka BJ, eds. *Transcultural Health Care: A Culturally Competent Approach*. 3rd ed. Philadelphia, PA: Davis; 2008:1–19.

QuickFacts. U.S. Census Bureau. *People QuickFacts*. Available at: QuickFacts.census.gov/qfd/states/00000.html. Accessed July 28, 2009.

Rando T. *Clinical Dimensions of Anticipatory Mourning*. Champaign, IL: Research Press; 2000.

Rando T. *Treatment of Complicated Mourning*. Champaign, IL: Research Press; 1993.

Richards M, Ersek M. *Communication at the End-of-Life. Palliative Care Resource Education Team (PERT) Train-the-Trainer Curriculum*. Seattle, WA: Swedish Medical Center; 2004.

Ritchie MA. Self-esteem and hopefulness in adolescents with cancer. *J Pediatr Nurs*. 2001;16:35–42.

Runyan BA. *AASLD Practice Guidelines: Management of Adult Patients with Ascites Due to Cirrhosis: An Update*. 2009. Available at: aasld.org/practiceguidelines/Documents/Bookmarked%20Practice%20Guidelines/Ascites%20Update6-2009.pdf. Accessed February 3, 2010.

Sheldon JE, Poleto MA. Personal and professional development. In: Ersek M, ed. *Hospice and Palliative Nursing Assistant Core Curriculum*. Pittsburgh, PA: Hospice and Palliative Nurses Association; 2009: 87–93.

Sorrentino S, Gorek B. *Mosby's Textbook for Long-Term Care Assistants*. 4th ed. St. Louis, MO: Mosby; 2003:76, 88–95.

Steele RG, Fitch MI. Coping strategies of family caregivers of home hospice patients with cancer. *Oncol Nurs Forum*. 1996;23(6):955–960.

Steele RG, Fitch MI. Needs of family caregivers of patients receiving home hospice care for cancer. *Oncol Nurs Forum*. 1996;23(5):823–828.

Stephenson PL, Draucker CB, Martsolf DS. The experiences of spirituality in the lives of hospice patients. *J Hosp Palliat Nurs*. 2003;5(1):51–58.

Stevenson L. The role and function of the interdisciplinary psychotherapeutic team in oncology care. In: Carroll-Johnson RM, Gorman LM, Bush NJ, eds. *Psychosocial Nursing Along the Cancer Continuum*. Pittsburgh, PA: ONS Press; 1998:277–284.

Storey P, Knight CF. *Hospice/Palliative Care Training for Physicians (UNIPACS 2, 2, 4, 6)*. 3rd ed. Chicago, IL: American Academy of Hospice and Palliative Medicine; 2008.

SUPPORT Principal Investigators. A controlled trail to improve care for seriously ill hospitalized patients. The study to understand prognoses and preferences for outcomes and risk of treatments (SUPPORT). *J Am Med Assoc*. 1995;274:1591–1598.

Taylor EJ. *Spiritual Care: Nursing Theory, Research, and Practice*. Upper Saddle River, NJ: Prentice-Hall; 2002.

Taylor EJ. Spiritual needs of patients with cancer and family caregivers. *Cancer Nurs*. 2003;26(4):260–266.

Taylor EJ. Spirituality and the cancer experience. In: Carroll-Johnson RM, Gorman LM, Bush NJ, eds. *Psychosocial Nursing Care along the Cancer Continuum*. 2nd ed. Pittsburgh, PA: Oncology Nursing Press; 2006:120–122.

Temkin-Greener H, Gross D, Kunitz SJ, Mukamel D. Measuring interdisciplinary team performance in a long-term care setting. *Med Care*. 2004;42(5):472–481.

Teno J, Lynn J, Wenger N, Phillips RS, Murphy DP, Connors AF. Advance directives for seriously ill hospitalized patients: effectiveness with the Patient Self-Determination Act and the SUPPORT intervention. *J Am Geriatrics Soc*. 1997;45:500–507.

The Joint Commission. *The Joint Commission Requirements*. Available at: www.jointcomission.org. Accessed February 2, 2010.

The SUPPORT Principal Investigators. A controlled trial to improve care for seriously ill patients. *JAMA*. 1995;274:1591–1598.

Tylor EB. *Primitive Culture* (Vols. 1 & 2). London, UK: Murray; 1871.

Vachon M, Sherwood C. Staff stress and burnout. In: Berger A, Portenoy R, Weissman D, eds. *Principles & Practice of Palliative Care & Supportive Oncology*. 2nd ed. Philadelphia, PA: Lippincott Williams & Wilkins; 2007:667–686.

Vachon ML. Psychosocial needs of patients and families. *J Palliat Care*. 1998;14(3):49–56.

Vaughn F. *The Inward Arc: Healing and Wholeness in Psychotherapy and Spirituality*. Boston, MA: New Science Library; 1986.

Victoria Hospice Society. *Palliative Performance Scale (PPSv2)*. 2001. Available at: palliative.info/resource_material/PPSv2.pdf. Accessed February 3, 2010.

Volker B. *Hospice and Palliative Nurses Practice Review*. 3rd ed. Dubuque, IA: Kendall Hunt Publishing; 1999:96–97.

Wadsworth B. *Piaget's Theory of Cognitive Development*. New York, NY: David McKay Co.; 1971.

Waller A, Caroline NL. *Handbook of Palliative Care in Cancer*. 2nd ed. Boston, MA: Butterworth-Heinemann; 2000.

Werth JL, Blevins D. *Decision-making Near the End of Life: Issues, Developments, and Future Directions*. New York, NY: Routhlede; 2009.

Wong DL. *Wong & Whaley's Clinical Manual of Pediatric Nursing*. 5th ed. St. Louis: Mosby; 2000.

Worden JW. *Children and Grief: When a Parent Dies*. New York, NY: The Guilford Press; 1996.

World Health Organization (WHO). *Report of a WHO Expert Committee: Cancer Pain Relief and Palliative Care*. WHO Technical Support Series, No. 804. Geneva: World Health Organization; 1986, 1990, 1996.

World Health Organization. *National Cancer Control Programs: Policies and Managerial Guidelines*. 2nd ed. 2002.

World Health Organization. *Cancer: Palliative Care*. Available at: www.who.int/cancer/palliative/en/. Accessed February 3, 2010.

World Health Organization. *WHO's Pain Ladder*. 2010. Available at: www.who.int/cancer/palliative/painladder/en/. Accessed February 8, 2010.

Yarbo CH, Frogge MH, Goodman M, eds. *Cancer Nursing: Principles and Practice*. 6th ed. Boston, MA: Jones and Bartlett Publishers; 2005.

Zoorenbos AZ, Schim SM. Cultural competence in hospice. *Am J of Hosp & Palliat Care*. 2004;21(1): 28–32.